Polyvinylpyrrolidone – Excipients for Pharmaceuticals

Volker Bühler

Polyvinylpyrrolidone Excipients for Pharmaceuticals

Povidone, Crospovidone and Copovidone

Springer

Volker Bühler
In den Weingärten 14
67157 Wachenheim/Weinstraße
Germany

ISBN 3-540-23412-8 Springer Berlin Heidelberg New York
Library of Congress Control Number: 2004112897

Springer is a part of Springer Science+Business Media

springeronline.com

Cover design: Design & Production, Heidelberg

Bühler: Polyvinylpyrrolidone Excipients for Pharmaceuticals

First Indian Reprint 2010

ISBN 978-81-8489-394-6

This edition is manufactured in India for sale only in India, Pakistan, Bangladesh, Nepal and Sri Lanka and any other country as authorized by the publisher.

This edition is published by Springer (India) Private Limited, (a part of Springer Science+Business Media), Registered Office: 3rd Floor, Gandharva Mahavidyalaya, 212, Deen Dayal Upadhyaya Marg, New Delhi – 110 002, India.

Printed at Saurabh Printers Pvt. Limited, Noida.

Contents

1 General notes on synthesis

1.1
Soluble polyvinylpyrrolidone (Povidone)

Modern acetylene chemistry is based on the work of Reppe. One of the many products of this work is N-vinylpyrrolidone (Fig. 1).

The first polymerization product of N-vinylpyrrolidone was soluble polyvinylpyrrolidone, which was patented in 1939. Fig. 2 and 3 show mechanisms of polymerization: free-radical polymerization in water using hydrogen peroxide as initiator or in 2-propanol using an organic peroxide as initiator [1, 141].

The mechanism for terminating the polymerization reaction makes it possible to produce soluble polyvinylpyrrolidone of almost any molecular weight.

Apart from the method of production in water shown in Fig. 2, it is also possible to conduct the polymerization in an organic solvent, e.g. 2-propanol, an with

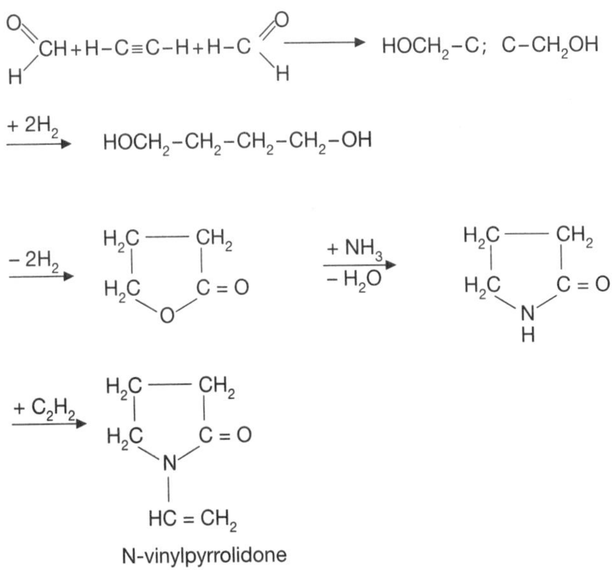

Fig. 1. Reppe's synthesis of N-vinylpyrrolidone (C_6H_9NO; Mr 111.1)

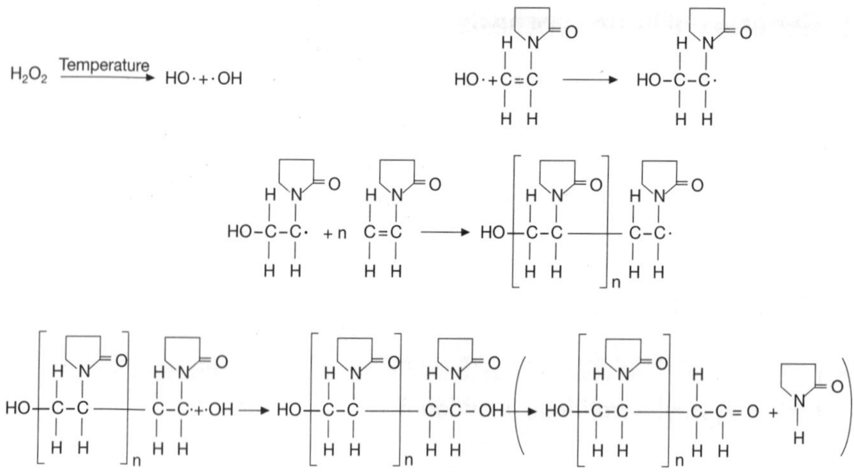

Fig. 2. The reaction mechanism for the radical polymerization of N-vinylpyrrolidone in water

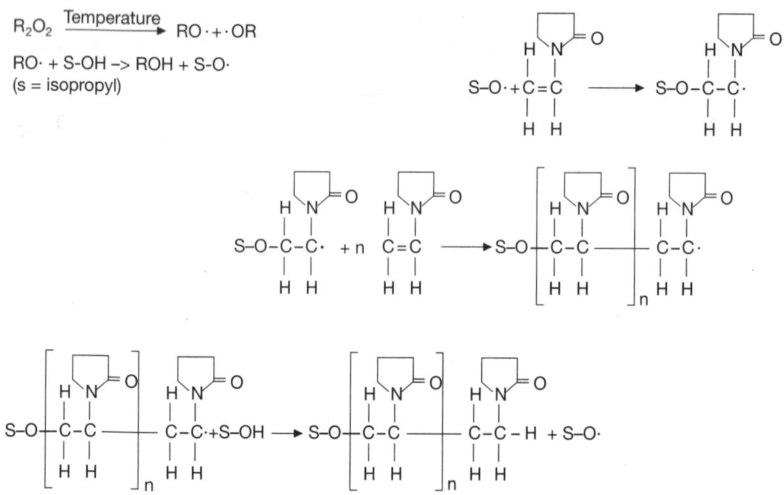

Fig. 3. The reaction mechanism for the radical polymerization of N-vinylpyrrolidone in 2-propanol

an organic peroxide as initiator (Fig. 3). This technology is used today in the production of low-molecular polyvinylpyrrolidone.

The low and medium-molecular weight grades of soluble polyvinylpyrrolidone are spray-dried to produce the pharmaceutical-grade povidone powders, while the high-molecular weight grades are roller-dried.

Soluble polyvinylpyrrolidone was first used during World War II as a blood-plasma substitute. Although it has excellent properties for this purpose, it has no longer been used for a number of decades. The organism does not metabolize the polymer, with the result that after parenteral administration, small quantities of high-molecular components may remain within the body. This problem does not exist with oral administration.

Today, soluble polyvinylpyrrolidone (povidone) is one of the most versatile and widely used pharmaceutical auxiliaries (see Section 2.4).

It is also used in the production of one of the most important topical disinfectants, povidone-Iodine.

1.2 Insoluble polyvinylpyrrolidone (Crospovidone)

Insoluble polyvinylpyrrolidone (crospovidone) is obtained by popcorn polymerization of N-vinylpyrrolidone [2], which yields a mainly physically crosslinked polymer [4–6]. The process is illustrated in Fig. 4 and uses either an alkali hydroxide at temperatures over 100°C, which yields some bifunctional monomer, or a small percentage of bifunctional monomer in water to initiate crosslinking of the polymer.

A comparison of the infrared spectra of the main physically crosslinked popcorn polymer obtained as shown in Fig. 4 and that of soluble polyvinylpyrrolidone shows practically no difference, while the infrared spectrum of a chemically crosslinked insoluble polyvinylpyrrolidone polymer prepared in the laboratory is quite different, which proves that the crosslinking in the crospovidone polymer is essentially of a physical nature.

Insoluble polyvinylpyrrolidone finds extensive applications in the pharmaceutical and beverage industries as a swelling popcorn polymer with selective adsorp-

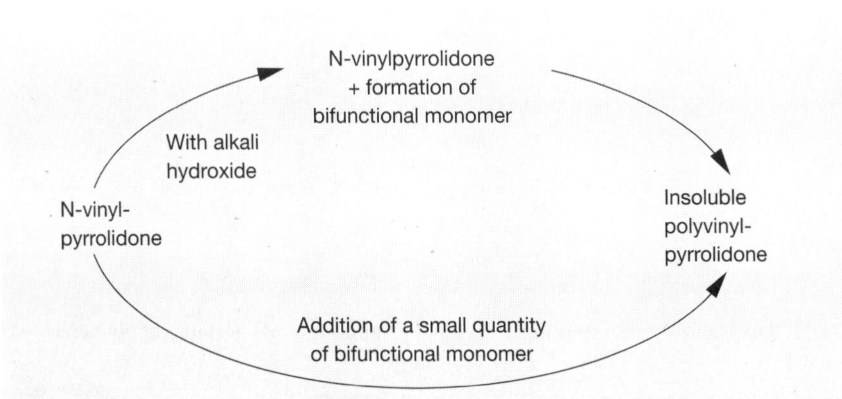

Fig. 4. Production processes for insoluble N-vinylpyrrolidone popcorn polymers (crospovidone)

tive properties. Its disintegration effect in tablets, its ability to hydrophylize insoluble active ingredients and to adsorb and form complexes are the main properties that make it useful as a pharmaceutical auxiliary. Today, crospovidone is regarded as one of the "superdisintegrants" for tablets.

Further, micronized crospovidone is of considerable significance as an active substance against diarrhoea in certain parts of the world. Micronized crospovidone grades of different bulk densities and different applications are available in the market.

1.3 Vinylpyrrolidone-vinyl acetate copolymer (Copovidone)

Water-soluble vinylpyrrolidone-vinyl acetate copolymer contains the two components in a ratio of 6 : 4. It is produced in the same way as soluble polyvinylpyrrolidone, by free-radical polymerization reaction with an organic peroxide as initiator (Fig. 5). As vinyl acetate is not soluble in water, the synthesis is conducted in an organic solvent such as 2-propanol.

Because of its vinyl acetate component, copovidone is somewhat more hydrophobic and gives less brittle films. This gives the product its favourable properties as a soluble binder and film-forming agent, particularly for solid dosage forms.

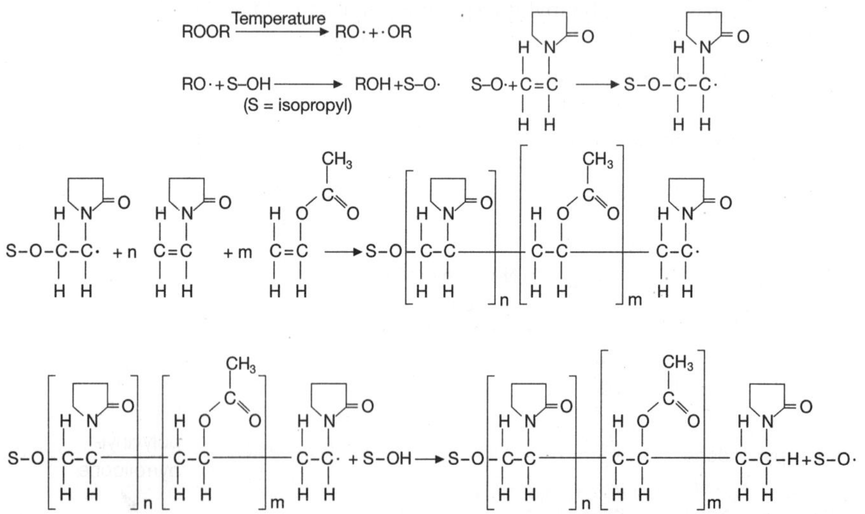

Fig. 5. Free-radical polymerization of vinylpyrrolidone-vinyl acetate copolymer (n +1) : m = 6 : 4

2 Soluble polyvinylpyrrolidone (Povidone)

2.1
Structure, product range and synonyms

Soluble polyvinylpyrrolidone is obtained by free-radical polymerization of vinylpyrrolidone in water or 2-propanol, yielding the chain structure of Fig. 6 [1, 141].

The current range of povidone consists of pharmaceutical grade products with different nominal K-values given in Table 1. All povidone grades are produced in according to the cGMP regulations.

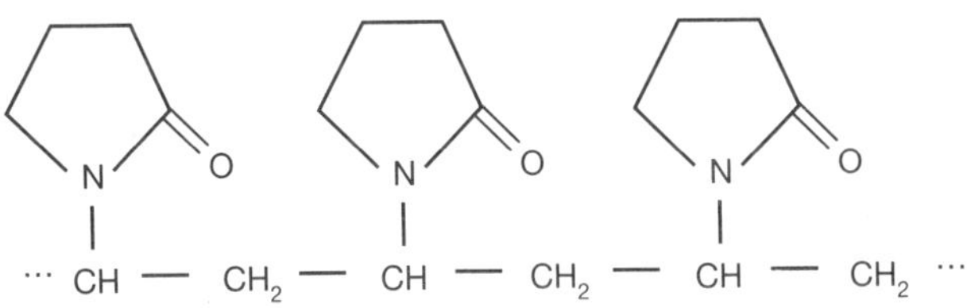

Fig. 6. Chemical structure of soluble polyvinylpyrrolidone (povidone) Mr $(111.1)_x$

Table 1. Povidone grades available in the market

Povidone grade	Trade names	Manufacturer
Povidone K 12*	Kollidon® 12PF	BASF
Povidone K 17*	Kollidon® 17PF, Plasdone® C-15	BASF, ISP
Povidone K 25	Kollidon® 25, Plasdone® K-25	BASF, ISP
Povidone K 30	Kollidon® 30, Plasdone® K-29/32	BASF, ISP
Povidone K 90	Kollidon® 90F, Plasdone® K-90	BASF, ISP
	Plasdone® K-90 D**, Plasdone® K-90 M**	ISP

* endotoxin or pyrogen free grades; ** D = densified, M = milled

Kollidon® is a registered trademark of BASF AG, Ludwigshafen, Germany
Plasdone® is a registered trademark of ISP Investments Inc., Wilmington, Delaware, USA

Table 2. Official names and abbreviations for soluble polyvinylpyrrolidone

Name/abbreviation	Origin/area of application
Povidone	Current valid Pharmacopoeias (e.g. USP 26, Ph.Eur. 5, JP 14)
Polyvidon(e)	Former editions of Pharmacopoeias (e.g. Ph.Fr. IX)
Povidonum	Pharmacopoeias (e.g. Ph.Eur. 5)
Polyvidonum solubile	Former edition of the DAC (1986)
Poly(1-vinyl-2-pyrrolidon)	Deutsches Arzneimittelgesetz 1984 § 10 (6)
PVP	General abbreviation, commercial name for cosmetics/technical grade

Spray drying technology is used in the production of all povidone grades with the exception of povidone 90. Because of its very high average molecular weight, it has to be dried on a roller.

Soluble polyvinylpyrrolidone is known under the names and abbreviations given in Table 2, most of which are specific to the pharmaceutical industry.

The CAS number of polyvinylpyrrolidone is 9003-39-8.

This book subsequently uses the name "Povidone".

2.2 Product properties

2.2.1 Description, specifications, pharmacopoeias

2.2.1.1 *Description*

All povidone grades are of pharmaceutical purity. They are free-flowing white or yellowish-white powders with different particle sizes (see Section 2.2.4).

The typical odour of the individual products depends on their method of synthesis and is therefore not the same for all the grades of povidone. Povidone K 25 and Povidone K 30, for instance, always have a typical amine or ammonia odour, as ammonia is used for neutralisation.

All the povidone types give aqueous solutions with very little taste.

2.2.1.2
Pharmacopoeial requirements, test methods

The products are tested according to the corresponding monographs for "Povidone" in the supplements of Ph.Eur. 5 and in USP 26. Their release for sale depends on fulfilment of the requirements of these monographs.

Table 3 contains the current pharmacopoeial requirements. The testing and guarantee of a particular microbial status and absence of pyrogens or endotoxins are not required by the pharmacopoeias in the povidone monographs.

The low-molecular grades povidone K 12 and povidone K 17 are tested for absence of bacterial endotoxins according to Ph.Eur. Method 2.6.14. A 6% solution in 0.9% sodium chloride solution is used. The validation of the endotoxin test (Ph.Eur. method 2.6.14) was done with povidone K 17 [609].

Low-molecular povidone can be polymerized in 2-propanol and in such case it contains the radical 2-propanol-vinylpyrrolidone adduct (hydroxy-methyl)-butylpyrrolidone as impurity (structure and determination see Section 2.3.3.8). The level of this impurity depends on the average molecular weight.

The products meet the ICH requirements on residual solvents according to Ph.Eur., 5.4: Only Class 3 solvents (2-propanol or formic acid) are likely to be present (<0.5%)

The microbial status can be determined according to Ph.Eur. methods 2.6.12 and 2.6.13 The usual limits (see Table 4) given in the European Pharmacopoeia apply to the categories 2 and 3A.

Table 3 see next page.

Table 4. Microbial purity requirements (Ph.Eur. 5, 5.1.4, Categories 2 + 3A)

- Max. 10^2 aerobic bacteria and fungi/g
- No Escherichia coli/g
- Max. 10^1 enterobacteria and other gramnegative bacteria/g
- No Pseudomonas aeruginosa/g
- No Staphylococcus aureus/g

Table 3. Pharmacopoeial requirements of povidone

	Povidone K 12	Povidone K 17	Povidone K 25	Povidone K 30	Povidone K 90
Clarity and colour (10% in water)	Clear and lighter than B6/BY6/R6	Clear and lighter than B6/BY6/R6	Clear and lighter than B6/BY6/R6	Clear and lighter than B6/BY6/R6	Clear and lighter than B6/BY6/R6
K-value (see 2.3.2.1)	10.2–13.8	15.3–18.4	22.5–27.0	27.0–32.4	81.0–97.2
Nitrogen content (%, see 2.3.3.6)	11.5–12.8	11.5–12.8	11.5–12.8	11.5–12.8	11.5–12.8
Water (K. Fischer, %)	≤ 5.0	≤ 5.0	≤ 5.0	≤ 5.0	≤ 5.0
pH (5% in water)	3.0–5.0	3.0–5.0	3.0–5.0	3.0–5.0	4.0–7.0
Vinylpyrrolidone (ppm, see 2.3.3.2)	≤ 10	≤ 10	≤ 10	≤ 10	≤ 10
Sulfated ash (%)	≤ 0.1	≤ 0.1	≤ 0.1	≤ 0.1	≤ 0.1
Aldehyde (%, see 2.3.3.3)	≤ 0.05	≤ 0.05	≤ 0.05	≤ 0.05	≤ 0.05
Heavy metals (ppm)	≤ 10	≤ 10	≤ 10	≤ 10	≤ 10
Hydrazine (ppm)	≤ 1	≤ 1	≤ 1	≤ 1	≤ 1
Peroxides (ppm H_2O_2)	≤ 400	≤ 400	≤ 400	≤ 400	≤ 400
2-Pyrrolidone (%, see 2.3.3.2)	≤ 3.0	≤ 3.0	≤ 3.0	≤ 3.0	≤ 3.0
Formic acid (%, see 2.3.3.4)	–	–	≤ 0.5	≤ 0.5	≤ 0.5
2-Propanol (%, see 2.3.3.4)	≤ 0.5	≤ 0.5	–	–	–
Organic volatile impurities (USP)	Passes test	Passes test	Passes test	Passes test	Passes test
Bacterial endotoxins (Ph.Eur. 5)*	= ≤0.1 I.U./mg	= ≤0.1 I.U./mg			

* monograph "Substances for pharmaceutical use"

Table 5. Countries in which povidone fulfil the requirements of the pharmacopoeias

Country	Pharmacopoeia
More than 30 european countries (Examples)	Ph.Eur. 5, Suppl. 4.7
Austria	ÖAB
Belgium	Ph.Belg.
France	Ph.Fr.
Germany	DAB
Great Britain	BP
Italy	F.U.
Netherlands	Ph.Ned.
Scandinavia	Ph.Nord.
Spain	F.E.
USA	USP 26
Japan (only Kollidon® 25, 30 and 90 F)	J.P. 14
Japan (only Kollidon® 17 PF)	JPE

2.2.1.3
Pharmacopoeias

Povidone complies with the harmonized monographs in the pharmacopoeias of the countries listed in Table 5. The list is not comprehensive.

2.2.2
Solubility, dissolution

One of salient features of povidone is its universal solubility, which extends from extremely hydrophilic solvents, such as water, to hydrophobic liquids, such as butanol.

Today, the use of organic solvents, such as methylene chloride or chloroform is severely restricted, but nevertheless, small quantities of organic solvents are still used by most pharmaceutical companies. The most commonly used are ethanol, propylene glycol or low-molecular polyethylene glycol. Povidone is miscible in practically all proportions in these solvents and in water, though, above a certain concentration, the solution obtained has a high viscosity (see Section 2.2.3).

Table 6 lists a number of solvents that are capable of forming solutions containing either more than 10% or not more than 1% of povidone. The solubility in acetone is 1–2%.

The dissolution behaviour and dissolution rate are typical for a polymer. It is recommended to add the powder slowly and in small portions to the solvent with vigorous stirring to ensure that it disperses and dissolves rapidly without forming lumps. Larger lumps dissolve rather slowly. This applies particularly to povidone K 90, as this high-molecular grade dissolves more slowly than the low-molecular grades.

Table 6. Solubility of povidone

More than 10% in:	Less than 1% in:
Water	
Diethylene glycol	Ethyl acetate
Methanol	Dioxane
Ethanol	Diethyl ether
n-Propanol	Pentane
Isopropanol	Cyclohexane
n-Butanol	Carbon tetrachloride
Chloroform	Toluene
Methylene chloride	Xylene
2-Pyrrolidone	Liquid paraffin
Polyethylene glycol 400	Cyclohexanol
Propylene glycol	
1,4-Butanediol	
Glycerol	
Triethanolamine	
Propionic acid	
Acetic acid	

The surface tension and the conductivity of solutions with surfactants is not affected by the addition of povidone [492, 616].

2.2.3 Viscosity, K-value

2.2.3.1 *Viscosity in water*

The viscosity of aqueous solutions of povidone depends on their average molecular weight. This can therefore be calculated from the viscosity, giving the viscosity-average molecular weight (see Section 2.2.6). Fig. 7 shows the very considerable differences in viscosity between solutions of the different povidones in water, as a function of their concentration. A 20% aqueous solution of povidone K 12 shows hardly any visible difference to pure water, while a 20% solution of povidone K 90 in water gives high viscosities until 5000 mPa·s.

Differentiations between the individual types of different molecular weight are made on the basis of their relative viscosity in water and their K-value, which can be calculated from the former according to the Ph.Eur. and USP monographs, "Povidone". The tolerance limits for the K-value given in Table 9 can similarly be calculated from the viscosity limits given in Table 7 using the methods given in these monographs.

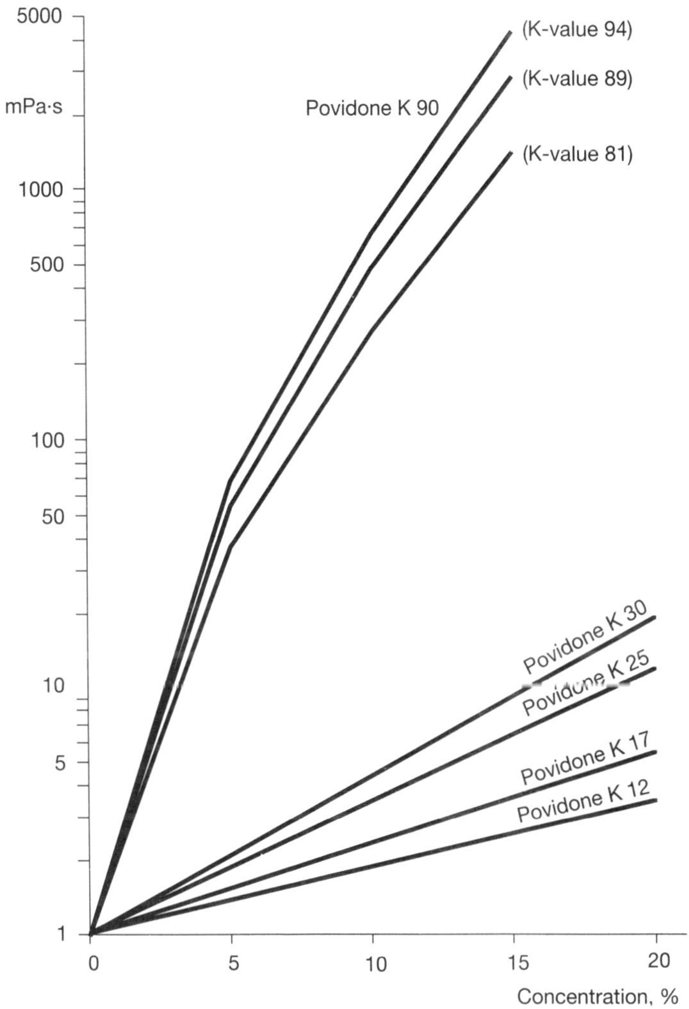

Fig. 7. Viscosity curves for the povidone grades in water (capillary viscometer, 25 °C)

Table 7. Relative viscosity values for povidone in water for calculating the K-value according to Ph.Eur. and USP (capillary viscometer, 25 °C)

Nominal K-value	Concentration	Relative viscosity USP and Ph.Eur. limits
12	5%	1.222–1.361
17	5%	1.430–1.596
25	1%	1.146–1.201
30	1%	1.201–1.281
90	1%	3.310–5.195

If the concentrations of the solutions are increased, the viscosity ranges become even greater, as can be seen from the values given in Table 8 for 10% (g/ml) solutions in water. These typical values have been taken from the former monograph "Lösliches Polyvidon" in Deutscher Arzneimittel-Codex 1986.

The viscosity, e. g. of povidone K 30 in water at concentrations up to 10%, is hardly affected by temperature (Fig. 8). At higher concentrations, however, the viscosity decreases rapidly with increasing temperature.

It was reported that most cations increase the viscosity and most of anions decrease the viscosity of povidone K 90 solutions [530]. Some polymers such as carragheenan show a synergistic viscosity increasing effect with the high-molecular povidone K 90.

It must be emphasized that the viscosity of povidone solutions is independent of their pH over a wide range. Only in extreme cases does this rule not apply: concentrated hydrochloric acid increases their viscosity; strong alkali precipitates povidone. However, it usually redissolves on addition of water.

Highly concentrated solutions of povidone K 90 demonstrate a certain degree of associative thickening and their viscosity is reduced by strong shear forces.

Table 8. Typical viscosity values for 10 % (g/ml) solutions of povidone in water at 20°C (DAC 1986)

Product	K-value range	Typical viscosity range
Povidone K 12	11–14	1.3–2.3 mPa s
Povidone K 17	16–18	1.5–3.5 mPa s
Povidone K 25	24–27	3.5–5.5 mPa s
Povidone K 30	28–32	5.5–8.5 mPa s
Povidone K 90	85–95	300–700 mPa s

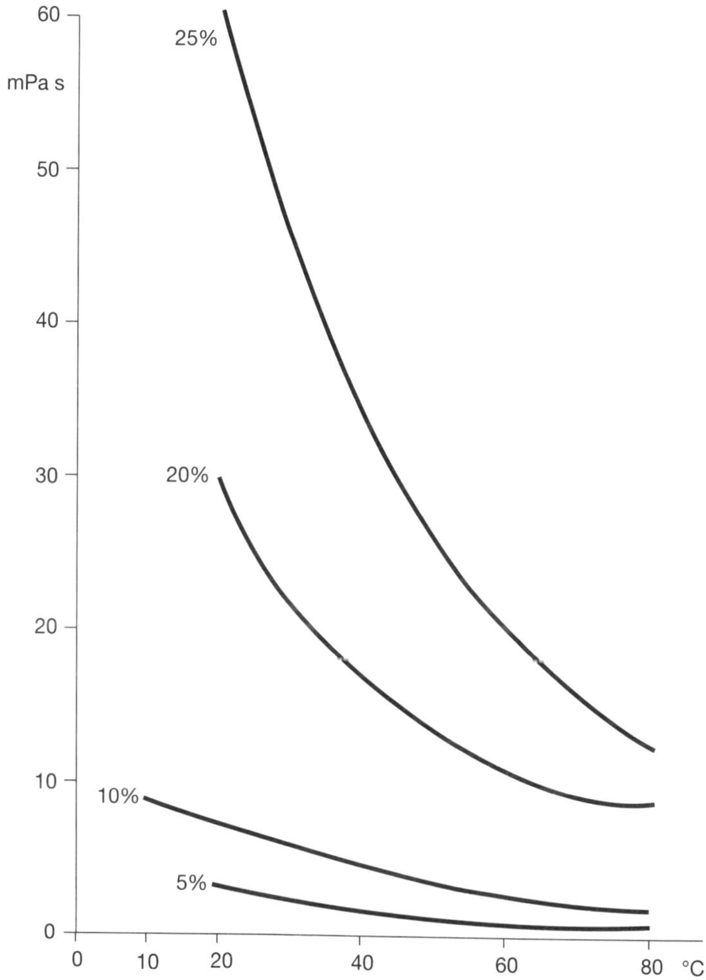

Fig. 8. The viscosity of different povidone K 30 solutions in water as a function of temperature

2.2.3.2
K-value

The average molecular weight of povidone is expressed in terms of the K-value in the pharmacopoeias valid in Europe, the USA and Japan [13]. It is calculated from the relative viscosity in water and always forms a part of the commercial name. The K-values specified in Section 2.2.1.2 are the ranges specified in the European Pharmacopoeia (Ph.Eur.). As can be seen from Table 9, the K-value ranges specified in the USP are identical. The USP and Ph.Eur. specify harmonized limits of 85–115% for nominal (= stated) K-values up to 15, while for nominal K-values

Table 9. Pharmacopoeia requirements for the K-values of povidone (calculated from Table 7)

Nominal K-value	USP and Ph.Eur. specification
12	10.2–13.8
17	15.3–18.4
25	22.5–27.0
30	27.0–32.4
90	81.0–97.2

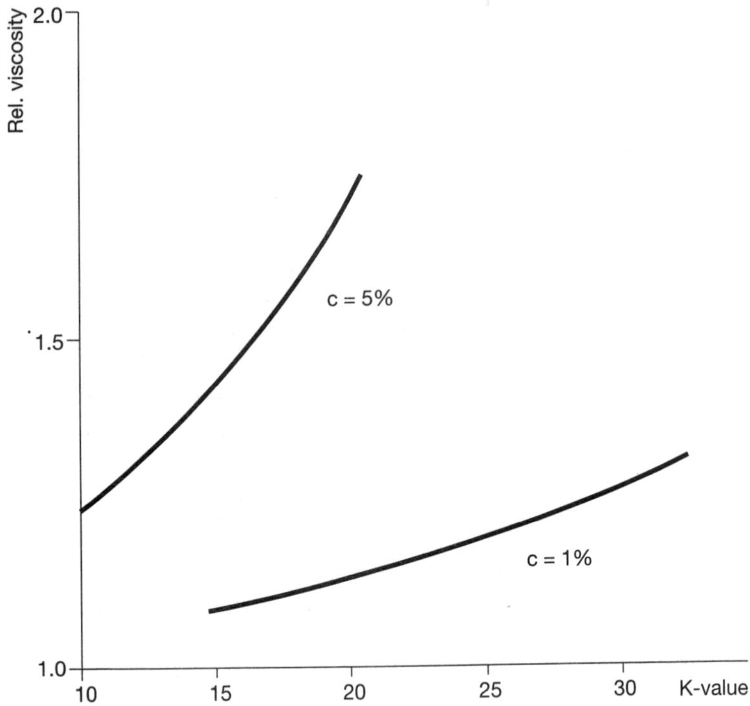

Fig. 9. Relative viscosity in water between K-values 10 and 33 [13]

above 15, they allow limits of 90–108% of the K-value. The values in Table 9 were calculated from the data in Table 7 (formula: see Section 2.3.2.1).

Figures 9 and 10 show the relative viscosity as a function of the K-value for 1% and 5% solutions in water.

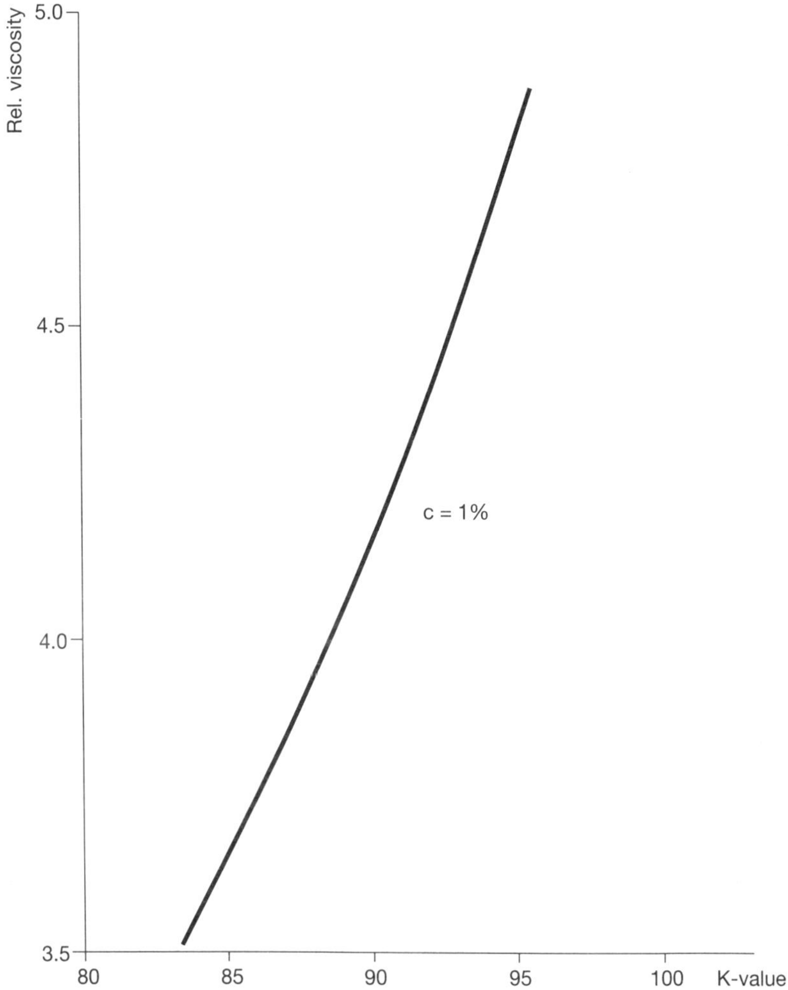

Fig. 10. Relative viscosity in water between K-values 83 – 95 [13]

2.2.3.3
Viscosity in alcohols

The viscosity of alcoholic solutions of povidone is significantly higher than that of aqueous solutions, as can be seen from the values in Table 10. The solvents most commonly used in tablet granulation, ethanol and 2-propanol, have been selected as examples.

The values given in Table 10 vary, of course, according to the K-value range of the individual product. Major deviations are found particularly with the high-molecular povidone K 90.

Table 10. Viscosity of 5 % organic solutions of povidone at 25 °C (typical values)

	Ethanol	Isopropanol
Povidone K 12	1.4 mPa s	2.7 mPa s
Povidone K 17	1.9 mPa s	3.1 mPa s
Povidone K 25	2.7 mPa s	4.7 mPa s
Povidone K 30	3.4 mPa s	5.8 mPa s
Povidone K 90	55.0 mPa s	90.0 mPa s

2.2.3.4
Intrinsic viscosity

The intrinsic viscosity of unfractionated povidone can be determined by various methods [212]. In Fig. 11, the intrinsic viscosity of povidone K 30 is determined by extrapolation to zero concentration of measurements at different concentrations, giving a value of 0.207 dl/g.

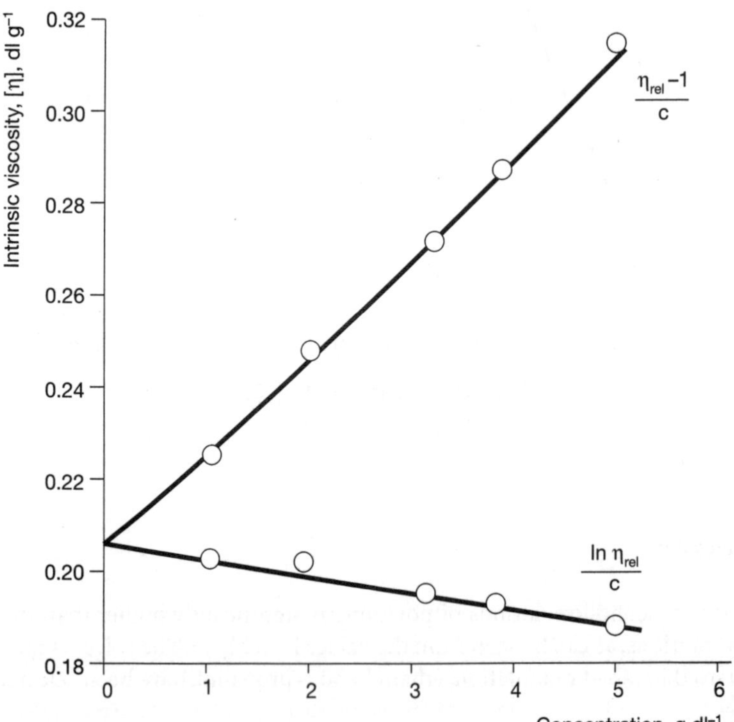

Fig. 11. Determination of the intrinsic viscosity [h] of povidone K 30 in water by extrapolation [212]

A simpler method for determining the intrinsic viscosity is to calculate it from the relative viscosity at a single concentration [16]:

$$[\eta] = \frac{\eta_{rel} - 1}{c + 0.28\, c\, (\eta_{rel} - 1)} \; (dl/g)$$

Figure 12 shows the intrinsic viscosity values obtained with this equation for povidone K 17, povidone K 25 and povidone K 30 at different concentrations in water [212]. Povidone K 17 is the only grade in which there is any significant variation in the viscosity between concentrations of 2% and 5%.
The values obtained in Fig. 11 by extrapolation agree well with the results in Fig 12.

A further method of determining the intrinsic viscosity from a single measurement is to calculate it from the K-value [223]:

$$[\eta] = 2.303\,(0.001\,K + 0.000075\,K^2)$$

The values obtained with this equation at different concentrations of povidone K 17, povidone K 25 and povidone K 30 largely agree with those in Fig. 12 [212].

A further method for determining the intrinsic viscosity from a measurement at a single concentration has been adopted in the former monographs of Japanese

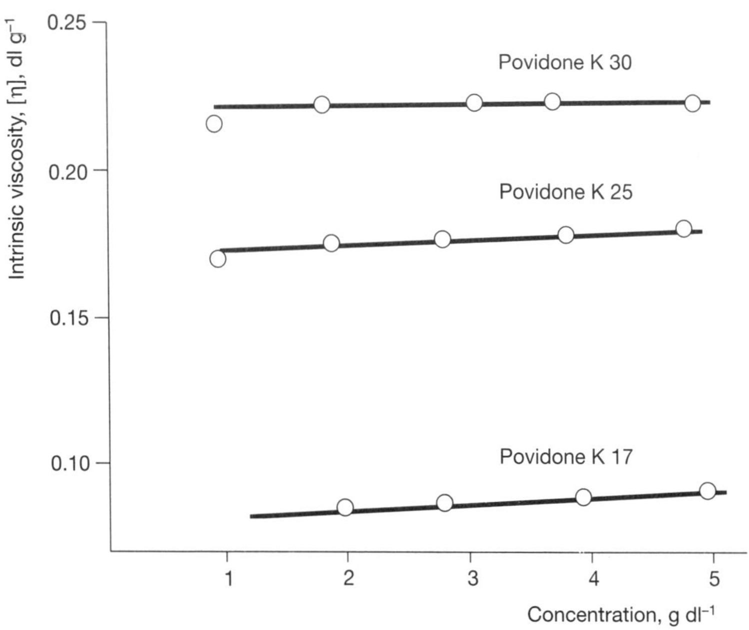

Fig. 12. Influence of the concentration of povidone K 17, povidone K 25 and povidone K 30 on their intrinsic viscosities, calculated according to [16]

Table 11. Intrinsic viscosity of povidone from Jap.Ph. XII

Povidone K 25	0.15 – 0.19
Povidone K 30	0.19 – 0.25
Povidone K 90	1.30 – 1.60

Pharmacopoeia (e. g. Jap.Ph. XII). It is based on the relative viscosity of a 1% solution of povidone in water and is calculated with the following equation:

$$\text{Intrinsic viscosity} = \frac{\ln \eta_{rel}}{\text{Sample concentration (g/dl)}}$$

Table 11 shows the ranges prescribed for the intrinsic viscosity in the former monographs of Jap.Ph. XII.

2.2.4 Particle size, particle structure, bulk density

2.2.4.1 *Particle size distribution*

In the manufacture of solid dosage forms, the particle size distribution of auxiliaries such as povidone can play a major role. This applies particularly to direct compression. However, the particle size of medium or high-molecular polymers also plays a role when they are used in liquid dosage forms. Table 12 lists a number of important factors related to the particle size, that must be considered in the manufacture of pharmaceuticals.

For these reasons, the fine fraction below 50 μm and the coarse fraction above 500 μm have been kept as small as possible in the non-micronized povidone types. Table 13 shows typical values for some individual povidone grades based on measurements with an air-jet screen.

Table 12. Important effects of particle size on the manufacture of pharmaceuticals

- A high proportion of fines spoils the flow properties.
- Fines produce dust.
- A high proportion of coarse particles leads to demixing.
- The coarse fraction is unevenly distributed in tablets.
- With high-molecular polymers, a large coarse fraction seriously delays dissolution.
- In direct compression, the coarse particles of a binder demonstrate a weaker binding effect.

Table 13. Typical sieve analysis of some povidone grades available on the market

Trade name	Fine fraction smaller than 74 µm	Coarse fraction larger than 297 µm
Kollidon® 25	less than 20 %	less than 5 %
Kollidon® 30	less than 20 %	less than 5 %
Kollidon® 90F	less than 10 %	less than 20 %
Plasdone® K-90	less than 5 %	less than 20 %
Plasdone® K-90D	less than 5 %	about 30 %
Plasdone® K-90M	about 30 %	less than 1 %

2.2.4.2
Particle structure

All povidone types with exception of roller dried povidone K 90 are spray dried powders and have therefore the typical particle structure of this technoloy.

Figure 13 shows an example of spray dried povidone. The structure are holow and mainly spherical particles. Figure 14 shows the completely different particle structure of the roller dried povidone K 90.

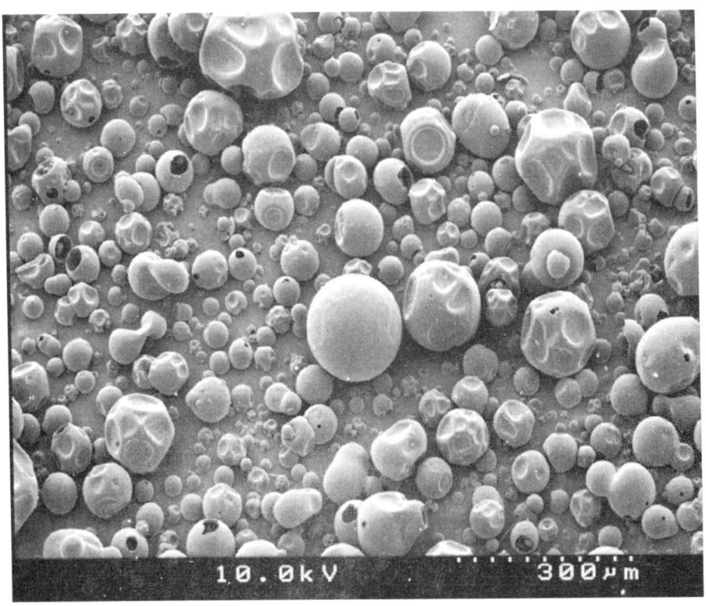

Fig. 13. Typical particle structure of spray-dried povidone (e.g. Kollidon® 30)

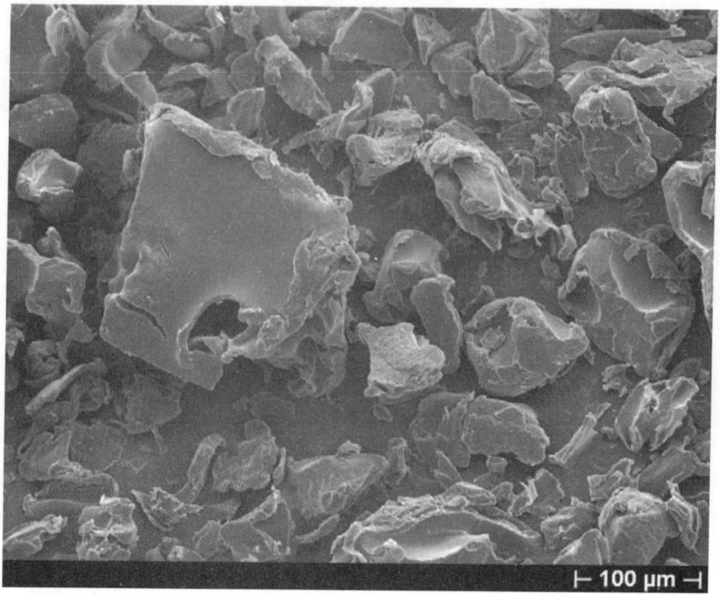

Fig. 14. Typical particle structure of roller-dried povidone K 90 (e.g. Kollidon® 90F)

2.2.4.3
Bulk density, tap density

The bulk densities of the spray-dried povidones are very similar. Table 14 gives typical values for the bulk and tap densities of the products on the market.

Table 14. Typical bulk and tap densities of povidone grades available on the market

Trade name	Bulk density (g/ml)	Tap density (g/ml)
Kollidon® 12PF	about 0.6	about 0.7
Kollidon® 17PF	about 0.45	about 0.55
Kollidon® 25	about 0.45	about 0.55
Kollidon® 30	about 0.45	about 0.55
Kollidon® 90F	about 0.45	about 0.6
Plasdone® C-15	about 0.34	about 0.44
Plasdone® K-25	about 0.34	about 0.44
Plasdone® K-29/32	about 0.34	about 0.43
Plasdone® K-90	about 0.29	about 0.39
Plasdone® K-90D	about 0.39	about 0.54
Plasdone® K-90M	about 0.56	about 0.72

2.2.5
Hygroscopicity

Povidone is a hygroscopic substance [140, 197], which can be an advantage or a disadvantage, depending on the application. When it is used as a binder or adhesive, it is an advantage, while for film-coating tablets it is a disadvantage. It has no effect on other applications, e.g. in solutions or suspensions. Figure 15 shows the moisture absorption curve as a function of relative humidity. It applies to all types of povidone and is one of the few parameters that is largely independent of the molecular weight. The increase in weight was determined after 7 days' storage at 25 °C over the solutions given in Table 15.

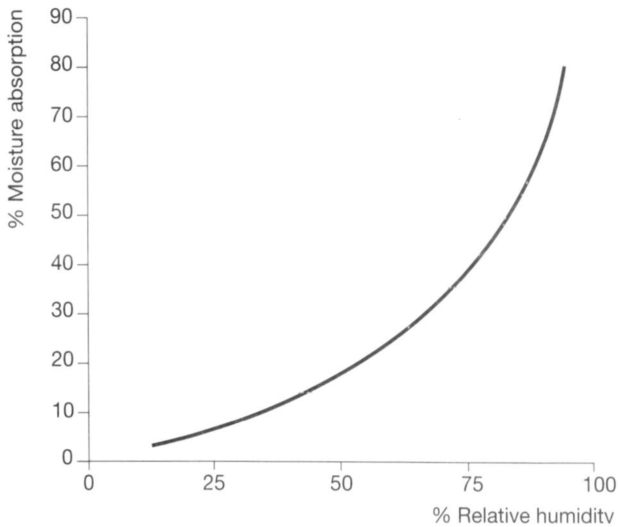

Fig. 15. Moisture absorption of povidone at 25 °C after 7 days

Table 15. Saturated solutions of salts for establishing constant relative humidity for the determination of moisture absorption

Salt	Relative humidity in the enclosed space above the solutions, %			
	20 °C	25 °C	30 °C	37 °C
Lithium chloride	12	11	11	11
Potassium acetate	24	23	23	23
Magnesium chloride	33	33	32	31
Potassium carbonate	44	43	42	41
Magnesium nitrate	53	52	52	51
Sodium nitrite	66	64	63	62
Sodium chloride	76	75	75	75
Potassium bromide	84	83	82	81
Potassium nitrate	94	93	92	91

The adsorption and desorption curves for povidone powders at room temperature are not the same. The two curves are shown for comparison in Fig. 16 [140].

As the absorption of water from the air is particularly critical in the film-coating of tablets, it was tested with cast films of povidone K 30 that contained 2.5% glycerol as a plasticizer. Figure 17 shows that a film of this type absorbs significantly less water within 72 hours at 85% relative humidity than the powder in Fig. 15. The absorption of moisture from the air is not completed within this period of time.

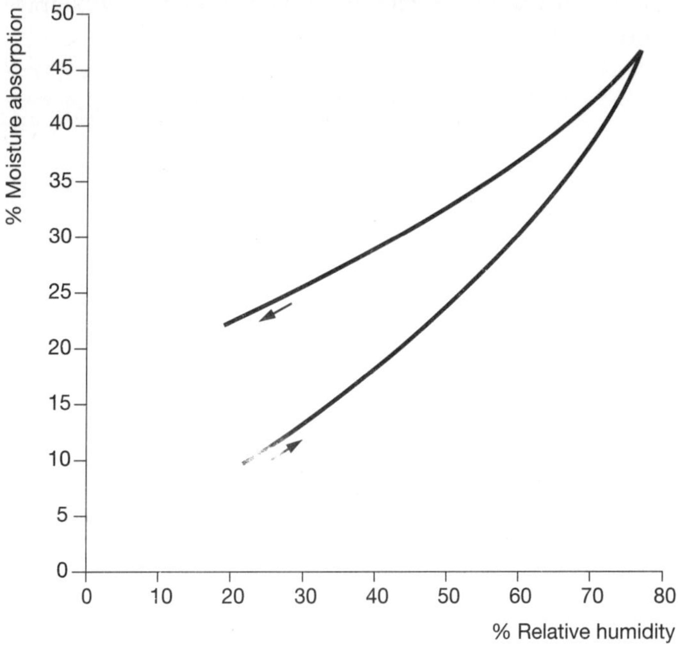

Fig. 16. Adsorption and desorption of atmospheric humidity by povidone powders at room temperature [140]

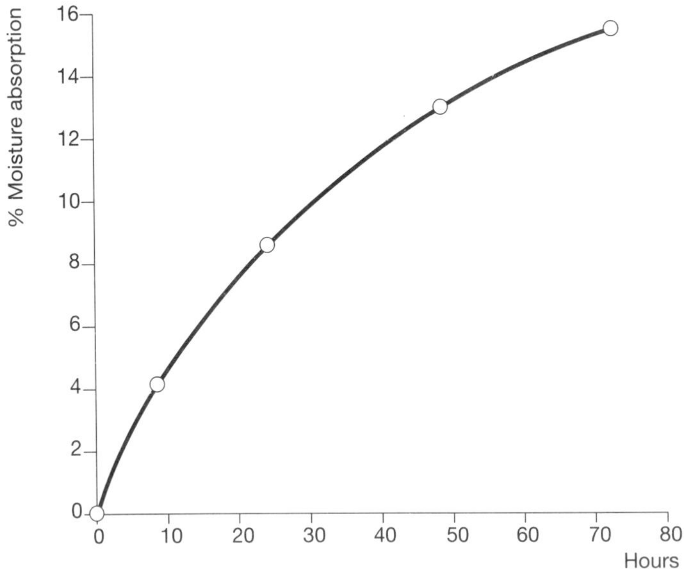

Fig. 17. Moisture absorbed by povidone K 30 films with 2.5 % glycerol over 72 hours at 25 °C and 85 % rel. humidity

2.2.6 Molecular weight

2.2.6.1 *Average molecular weight*

The average molecular weight of a polymer can be viewed and measured in three different ways [14, 212] as indicated in Table 16 below.

Table 16. Average molecular weights of polymers and their methods of determination

Type of average molecular weight	Symbol	Method of determination
Weight-average	$\bar{M}w$	Light scattering, ultracentrifuge
Number-average	$\bar{M}n$	Osmometry, membrane filtration
Viscosity-average	$\bar{M}v$	Viscosity

As these methods of determining the average molecular weight are relatively complicated, for povidone it is expressed in terms of the K-value, in accordance with the European and U.S. Pharmacopoeias (see also Section 2.2.3.2).

Figure 18 shows the relationship between the K-value and the average molecular weight $\overline{M}w$, determined by light scattering. A similar graph with the average molecular weight $\overline{M}v$ is given in the Section 2.3.2.2.

The weight-average of the molecular weight, $\overline{M}w$ is determined by methods that measure the weights of the individual molecules. The measurement of light scattering has been found to be the most suitable method for povidone [212]. Values determined by this method are given in Table 17. Recent results do not always agree well with older results, as the apparatus used has been improved significantly over the years. The products themselves have not changed, however.

The number-average of the molecular weight, $\overline{M}n$ is determined by methods that measure the number of molecules. This value is very seldom determined or published for povidone. Table 17 shows some older values.

The viscosity-average of the molecular weight, $\overline{M}v$ has attracted greater interest recently, as it can be calculated direct from the relative viscosity, the intrinsic viscosity or the K-value (see Section 2.3.2.2). Table 18 shows typical viscosity-average values for the different povidone types.

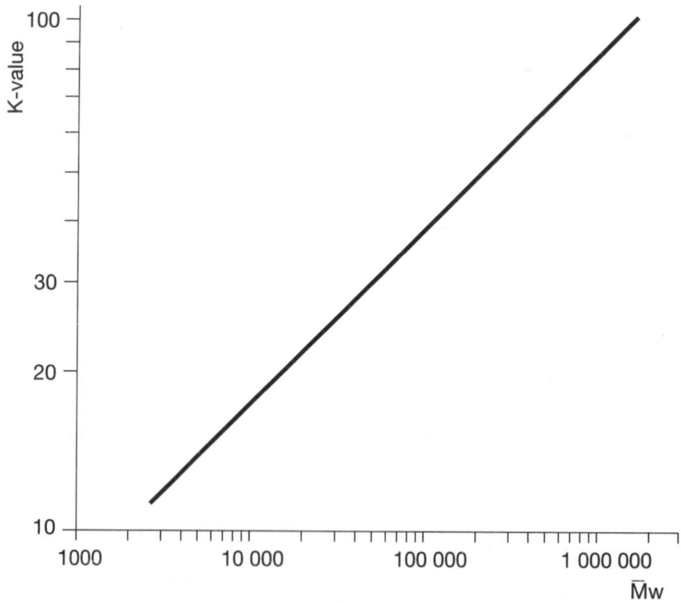

Fig. 18. K-value versus average molecular weight, $\overline{M}w$ determined by light scattering

Table 17. Weight and number-averages of the molecular weights of povidone

Kollidon grade	Weight-average (measured after 1980)	Weight-average (measured before 1980)	Number-average (older determinations)
Povidone K 12	2 000 – 3 000	2 500	1 300
Povidone K 17	7 000 – 11 000	9 000	2 500
Povidone K 25	28 000 – 34 000	25 000	6 000
Povidone K 30	44 000 – 54 000	40 000	12 000
Povidone K 90	1 000 000 – 1 500 000	700 000	360 000

Table 18. Viscosity-average values of the molecular weight, $\overline{M}v$ for povidone, calculated from the K-value [212]

	$\overline{M}v$ calculated from the nominal K-value	$\overline{M}v$ calculated from the K-value range given in Ph.Eur.
Povidone K 12	3 900	2 600 – 5 500
Povidone K 17	9 300	7 100 – 11 000
Povidone K 25	25 700	19 300 – 31 100
Povidone K 30	42 500	31 700 – 51 400
Povidone K 90	1 100 000	790 000 – 1 350 000

2.2.6.2
Molecular weight distribution

Polymers do not consist only of molecules of the same molecular weight, they consist of molecules with a range of molecular weights with, in the ideal case, a Gaussian distribution.

Gel permeation chromatography:
The molecular weight distribution of povidone can best be determined with the aid of high-performance gel permeation chromatography. Figure 19 gives a qualitative comparison between povidone K 17 and povidone K 30 in a gel permeation chromatogram marked at a molecular weight of 35 000.

Figure 20 shows the integral curve for a gel permeation chromatogram of povidone K 17, which gives a quantitative evaluation. The chromatograph was calibrated with povidone calibration fractions with sharply defined molecular weight ranges between 20 000 and 44 000. The curve shows that the cumulative percentage with a molecular weight greater than 35 000 is less than 5% for povidone K 17.

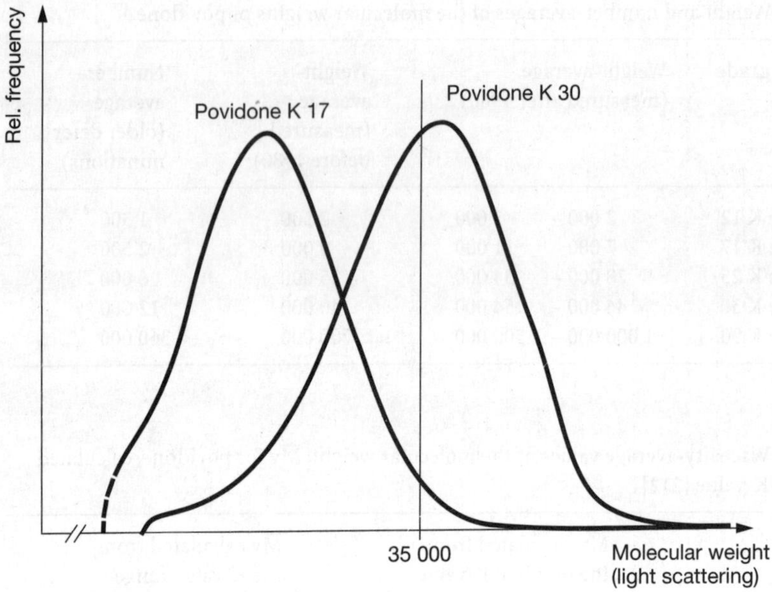

Fig. 19. Qualitative comparison of the molecular weight distributions of povidone K 17 and povidone K 30. Gel permeation chromatogram marked at a molecular weight of 35 000

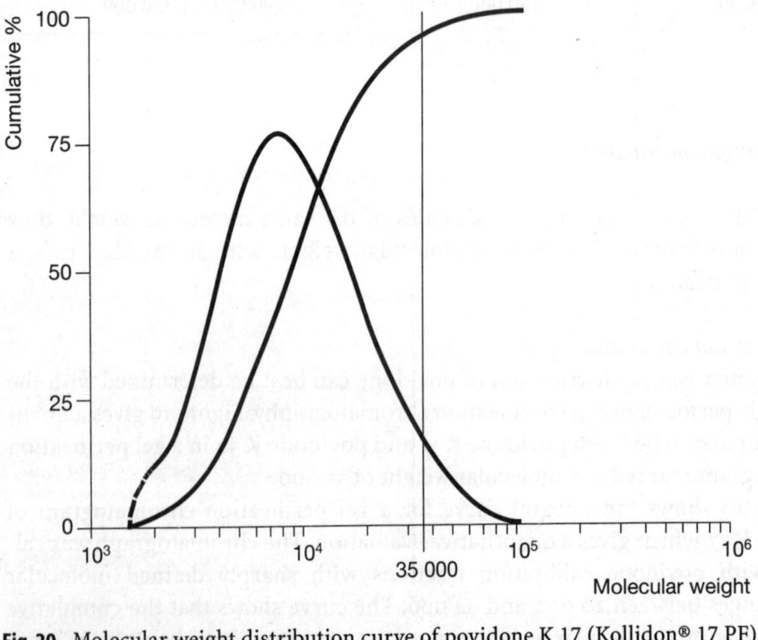

Fig. 20. Molecular weight distribution curve of povidone K 17 (Kollidon® 17 PF) with integral curve, determined by GPC

Light scattering:
A method suitable for the determination of the molecular weight distribution is the dynamic light scattering. The results are completely identical with the results obtained by the gel permeation chromatography because the method is not so sensitive for the low molecular weight part. But the reproducibility is better.

Fractionation:
A further means of obtaining information on the distribution of molecular weights in povidone is fractionation. This technique is very imprecise and gives only the proportions above and below a particular molecular weight. It is based on the difference in solubility of molecules of different sizes in certain solvents and their mixtures, e.g. water and isopropanol or ether.

This fractionation method has been adopted by the former Japanese Pharmacopoeia as a means of characterizing the high and low-molecular components of povidone. Certain combinations of water, isopropanol and acetone have been selected for this purpose and limits that have been established empirically are shown in Table 19.

Diafiltration:
In special cases, diafiltration with calibrated membranes can also be used to determine the proportions above and below a particular molecular weight. However, extensive testing has shown that the variations in the results are too great for the method to be readily reproducible, because of differences in pore size from one membrane to another and because of changes in the properties of the membranes after repeated use.

Electrophoresis:
Electrophoresis has also been described in the literature as a technique for determining the molecular weight distribution of povidone [377].

Table 19. Limits for the low and high-molecular components of povidone according to Jap.Ph. XII (former monographs)

Product	Low-molecular fraction	High-molecular fraction
Povidone K 25	max. 15%	max. 20%
Povidone K 30	max. 15%	max. 20%
Povidone K 90	max. 20%	–

2.2.7
Complexation, chemical reactions

2.2.7.1
Complexation

Because of its chemical structure, povidone forms chemical complexes with a number of substances, including pharmacologically active substances [7, 8, 44 c, 99, 103, 106, 179, 220]. Both the solubility and the stability of these complexes vary greatly. They almost always dissolve more readily or more quickly in water than the pure drug. Detailed information on the increase in solubility for individual active substances is given in Sections 2.4.3 and 2.4.5.

The only known exceptions, i.e. substances that become less soluble or even precipitate, are polyphenols, e.g. tannin, and hexylresorcinol [10, 108]. In general, all complexes with povidone are formed only under acidic conditions and are unstable and can decompose in the alkaline pH range. Typical examples are cobalt [388] and the disinfectant, povidone-iodine [9] in which all the iodine, with the exception of a few ppm of free iodine, is complexed (Fig. 21).

In systematic investigations into the dependence of complex formation on structure, no difference was found between soluble polyvinylpyrrolidone (povidone) and insoluble polyvinylpyrrolidone (crospovidone) for complexes with organic compounds [192].

The complex formation constant can be determined by a number of methods. The most important physical methods are based on adsorption tests, chromatography and dialysis. Table 20 lists the constants for a series of substances, mainly drugs, in 0.1 N hydrochloric acid.

Many further investigations into the formation of complexes by povidone with drugs have been described [e.g. 158, 179]. One of the methods used is differential scanning calorimetry [406 a–c], though this gives little information on the properties of the complex relevant to pharmaceutical technology. Sections 2.4.3 and 2.4.5 list a large number of publications of interest to the pharmaceutical technologist. In normal concentrations, the bonds that drugs form with povidone are comparable with those it forms with other auxiliaries in solid dosage forms, e. g.

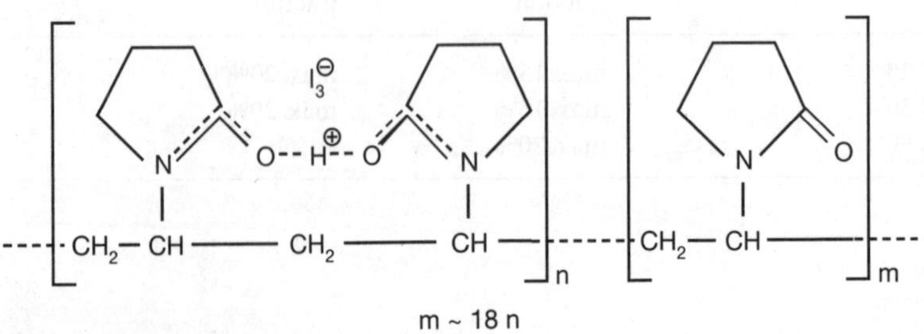

Fig. 21. Povidone-iodine complex

Table 20. Complex formation constants (l/mol) of a number of drugs and other substances with povidone [192]

Substance	Complex formation constant (l/mol) Sorption	Chromatography	Dialysis
Acetaminophen (= paracetamol)	< 1	< 1	1.5
Acetylsalicylic acid	< 1	< 1	0.7
Benzocaine	< 1	–	–
Benzoic acid	< 1	< 1	0.9
Chloramphenicol	*	*	0.4
Methotrimeprazine	4.6	5.2	3.2
Methylparaben	2.6	< 1	1.8
Phenol	< 1	< 1	0.8
Resorcinol	1.3	2.2	2.4
Riboflavin	< 1	–	–
Salicylamide	1.6	1.5	1.3
Salicylic acid	1.7	1.1	1.5
Sorbic acid	< 1	< 1	0.5
Sulfamoxole	*	*	0.3
Sulfathiazole	< 1	< 1	0.4
Tannic acid	> 1000	> 1000	–
Trimethoprim	*	*	0.2

* Not measurable

corn starch, cellulose and carboxymethyl cellulose [160]. However, the efficacy of certain preservatives, e.g. thiomersal, is affected, if there is a great excess of povidone [7, 11].

The influence that complexation can have on the absorption of an active substance by the body can be estimated with the aid of Fig. 22, if the concentration of povidone and the complexation constant are known [192].

The use of Fig. 22 in practice is illustrated in the following example: in a 4% aqueous solution of povidone K 90, it was found by ultrafiltration that 48.1% of the salicylic acid was complexed [179]. If these values are applied to Fig. 22, a complexation constant of about 2.9 l/mol is obtained. Even if high values for gastrointestinal povidone concentration, e.g. 0.5 g/l are taken, the complexed proportion of salicylic acid is less than 1% and can therefore be ignored.

As all the pharmaceutically active substances, apart from tannin, that have been checked to date have shown complexation constants of less than 10 l/mol, the above example for salicylic acid can be applied to almost all drugs. Complexation is widely used in pharmaceutical technology (Table 21).

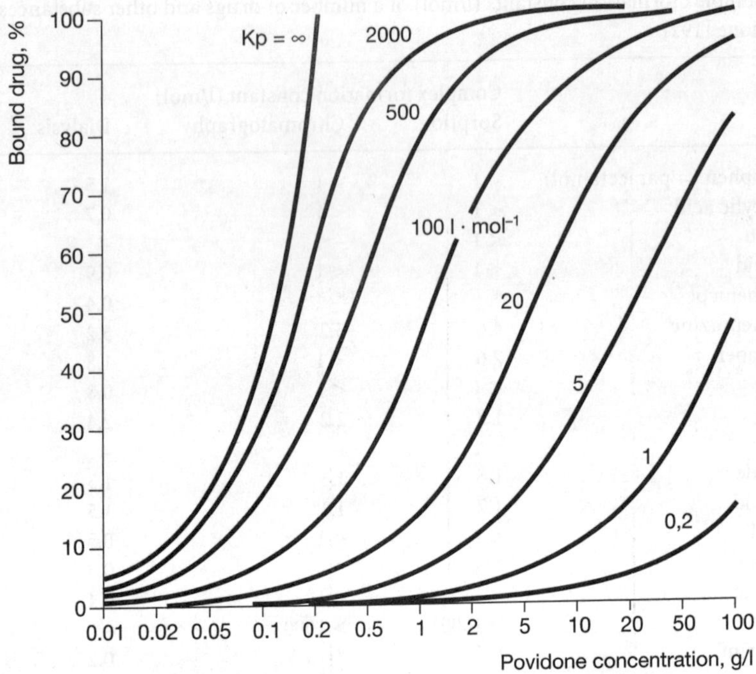

Fig. 22. Curves of drug complexation by povidone against povidone concentration for different complexation constants, Kp

Table 21. Use of the complexation of drugs with povidone in pharmaceutical technology

1. Improvement of the solubility of the drug in liquid dosage forms (Section 2.4.5)

   Examples: antibiotics, iodine, acetaminophen, sulfonamides

2. Acceleration of the dissolution rate of the drug from solid dosage forms (Section 2.4.3)

   Examples: dihydroergotamine, nabilone, nifedipine

3. Reduction of the toxicity of drugs (Section 2.4.8.4)

   Examples: iodine, oxytetracycline, endotoxins (of microbiological origin)

2.2.7.2
Further chemical interactions

Povidone can become insoluble as a result of crosslinking, particularly at higher temperatures, if it is combined with strongly alkaline substances such as lithium carbonate or sodium hydroxide [141]. In extreme cases, this could result in an increase in viscosity in liquid dosage forms or delayed bioavailability in tablets and capsules [217].

Povidone contains peroxides within the limits of the specification, though the content can increase in the course of storage. This can interfere with certain active substances such as ergot alkaloids and diagnostics.

2.2.8
Osmotic pressure, sterilization by filtration (Low-molecular povidone)

2.2.8.1
Osmotic pressure

The osmotic pressure of solutions is of particular importance with parenteral administration. (In the case of the human blood serum it is about 7.5 bar at 37 °C.) It is not very affected by the molecular weight and the concentration of povidone. The simplest method for determining the osmotic pressure uses the Van't Hoff equation.

The osmotic pressure values given in Table 23 were obtained for 10% solutions of low-molecular povidones in water, using the equation given in Table 22. These values apply to pure povidone. As povidone contains only traces of impurities, e.g. 1 ppm vinylpyrrolidone, the osmotic pressure is hardly affected. This is confirmed by comparing the values measured for povidone K 17 with those calculated, in Table 23. The osmotic pressure calculated for a solution containing 1 ppm vinylpyrrolidone is given for reference.

Table 22. Van't Hoff equation for calculating osmotic pressure, P

$$P = \frac{c \cdot R \cdot T}{Mn} \quad \text{(bar)}$$

c = concentration in g/l
R = gas constant 0.0821 l bar/degree
T = absolute temperature, °K
$\bar{M}n$ = number average of the molecular weight

Table 23. Osmotic pressure of low-molecular povidone solutions: calculated according to Table 22, and measured

Product	Concentration in water	Osmotic pressure (calculated)	Osmotic pressure (measured)
Povidone K 12	5%	ca. 1 bar	–
Povidone K 12	10%	ca. 2 bar	–
Povidone K 17	5%	ca. 0.5 bar	0.53 bar
Povidone K 17	10%	ca. 1 bar	1.06 bar
Vinylpyrrolidone	1 ppm	0.0002 bar	

2.2.8.2
Sterilization by filtration

It is important that injection solutions that contain low-molecular povidone can be sterilized by filtration. The feasibility of filtering these solutions is mainly determined by the concentration of these povidone grades. The viscosity evidently plays a subordinate role, as this is always less than 5 mPa s for povidone K 17 up to a concentration of 15% in water. With povidone K 12 it is even lower (see Section 2.2.3.1). Taking a batch of Kollidon® 17 PF as an example, it can be seen from Fig. 23 that the filtration time depends very much on the concentration. The

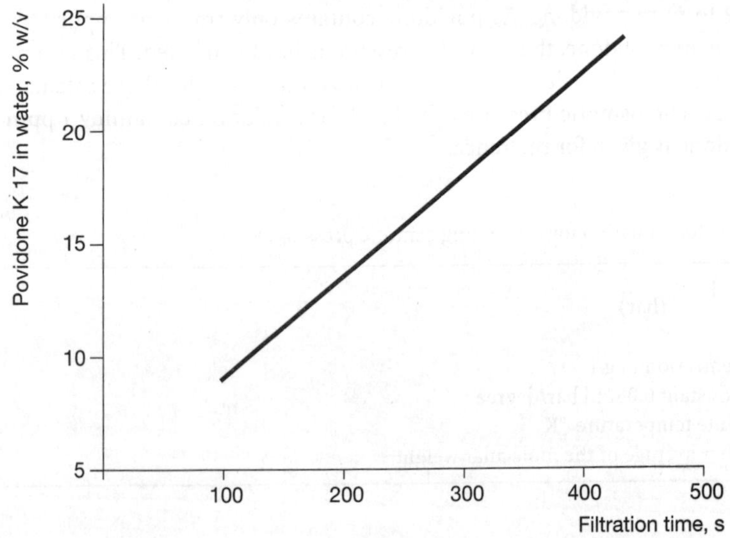

Fig. 23. Influence of the concentration of povidone K 17 (Kollidon® 17 PF) in water on the filtration time through a 0.45 μm filter of 47 mm diameter (500 ml solution, vacuum 90 mbar, room temperature)

results are based on laboratory measurements on 500 ml of solution under a vacuum of 90 mbar.

2.2.9
Stability, storage

2.2.9.1
Stability of the pure products

All types of povidone, with exception of povidone K 90, have very good storage stability in the pure form. Table 24 lists the minimum stabilities in the original sealed container at room temperature when these are stored and tested according to the requirements of the pharmacopoeias (see Section 2.2.1.2). Recently some povidone grades are commercialized with hermetically sealed aluminium-PE inliners under nitrogen and vacuum to increase the long term stability. This is mainly of interest for povidone K 90.

The lower stability of povidone K 90, compared with the other grades, is due to a slow decrease in the K-value. All the other parameters change just as little over a period of years, as those of other grades. If povidone K 90 is stored under cool conditions or if the original packaging never was opened the K-valuc decreases much less und the peroxides level remains much lower.

In the presence of atmospheric oxygen, the peroxide content of all the types of povidone grades slowly increases, but remains below the value of 400 ppm, calculated as H_2O_2, specified in Ph.Eur., within the storage periods given in Table 24.

The influence on the povidone powders of sterilization with gamma radiation was determined on a batch of Kollidon® 17 PF. Table 25 shows that this form of sterilization does not change either the molecular weight or the molecular weight distribution.

Table 24. Minimum stability ("retest date") of povidone stored in the original containers (max. 25°C, Ph.Eur. and USP requirements)

Product	Minimum shelf life
Povidone K 12	More than 3 years
Povidone K 17	More than 3 years
Povidone K 25	More than 3 years
Povidone K 30	More than 3 years
Povidone K 90	More than 1 or 2 years*

* depending on the packaging

Table 25. Influence of gamma radiation on the molecular weight of povidone K 17 powder (Kollidon® 17 PF)

Radiation	Molecular weight Number average	 Weight average
None	4700	9500
10 kGy	4700	9500
25 kGy	4700	9600
50 kGy	4700	9600

2.2.9.2
Stability in solid dosage forms

Because of the good stability of povidone on its own, its stability in solid dosage forms is usually also good.

Up to now, only isolated cases have become known, in which the stability of povidone has deteriorated in solid dosage forms. One of these is the combination with strongly alkaline substances, which can cause the polymer to crosslink, particularly at elevated temperatures [141]. As the example of lithium carbonate has shown many years ago, this can lead to a reduction in bioavailability [217].

The peroxides formation was studied in tablets based on microcrystalline cellulose, magnesium stearate and 5% povidone K 30 at room temperature. The level of peroxides decreased continuously during 2 years to less than 25% of the initial value in all tablets obtained by direct compression or by wet granulation.

2.2.9.3
Stability in liquid dosage forms

A change in colour is sometimes observed in aqueous solutions of povidone grades after storage or heating, e.g. during sterilization. The yellow or brown-yellow colour is formed as a result of oxidation and can therefore be prevented by the addition of a suitable antioxidant.

The change in colour of a 20% solution of povidone K 17 (Kollidon® 17 PF) in water was from a slight yellow tint (Yellow 7 according to Ph.Eur.) to stronger yellow (Yellow 4) after thermal sterilization at 120–121 °C for 20 min. The addition of 0.2% of sodium bisulfite provided excellent colour stabilization. Ascorbic acid cannot be used as an antioxidant as it undergoes hydrolysis itself, giving rise to an even darker yellow-brown colour.

A 10% solution of povidone K 30 in water can be stabilized by the addition of 0.5% of cysteine or 0.02% of sodium sulfite against discolouration by heat sterilization. The Table 26 shows in a storage test of aqueous solution of povidone that the application of nitrogen is not effective because it contains always some residues of oxygen. The formation of peroxides, free vinylpyrrolidone or turbity is no problem and the influence of the pH is negligible.

Table 26. Storage of solutions of 10% of povidone in water at different pH's in the dark during 3 months at 40 °C (Ph.Eur. methods)

Parameter	pH	Initial values	After storage under air	After storage under nitrogen	After storage (Addition of 0.5% cysteine
Povidone K 30 (Kollidon® 30)					
Colour (B = brown, Y = yellow)	2.0 6.4 9.0	B 6–7 B 6–7 B 6–7	Y 4–5 Y 3–4 BY 4–5	Y 3–4 Y 3–4 Y 4–5	BY 5–6 Y 5–6 B 6–7
Clarity*	2.0–6.4 9.0	1.3 FTU 1.5 FTU	<1 FTU 1.3 FTU	<1 FTU 1.3 FTU	<1 FTU 1.1 FTU
Peroxides	2.0 6.4–9.0	70 ppm 30 ppm	20 ppm 20 ppm	<20 ppm <20 ppm	<20 ppm <20 ppm
Vinylpyrrolidone	2.0–9.0	<1 ppm	<1 ppm	<1 ppm	<1 ppm
Povidone K 90 (Kollidon® 90F)					
Colour (B = brown, Y = yellow)	2.0 6.4	B 6–7 B 6–7	BY 6–7 BY 5–6	BY 5–6 BY 4–5	BY 6–7 B 7
Clarity*	2.0 6.4	1.0 FTU 1.3 FTU	1.1 FTU 1.4 FTU	1.6 FTU 1.3 FTU	1.2 FTU 2.7 FTU
Peroxides	2.0	180 ppm	180 ppm	140 ppm	<20 ppm
Vinylpyrrolidone	!2.0–6.4	<1 ppm	<1 ppm	<1 ppm	<1 ppm

* The definition of the clarity like water according to Ph.Eur. corresponds to & 2.0 FTU (= Formazine Turbity Unit)

Similar results were found with respective solutions of the low-molecular povidone Kollidon® 17 PF.

If sodium bisulfite is to be used as an antioxidant in parenteral preparations, the legal situation in the respective country must be considered.

2.2.9.4 *Stability of the molecular weight in liquid dosage forms after thermal sterilization and storage*

As the molecular weight determines many of the properties of povidone that affect its use, it is worth knowing that it is not changed by storage or heating. In solutions, a change in the relative viscosity most readily reveals an increase or decrease in the average molecular weight. Extensive tests have been conducted with solutions (Table 27), in which the viscosity was measured to determine the influence of sterilization on the average molecular weight (Table 28). No change was found even at pH as high as 10.

The influence of storage on the average molecular weight was tested by keeping the solutions in Table 27 for four weeks at 60°C and 70°C. Even after this accelerated storage test, no increase or decrease in the mean molecular weight of povidone K 12 and povidone K 17 could be measured.

To determine the influence of storage on the molecular weight distribution, gel permeation chromatography separations were conducted on new and up to 5-year-old, commercially available pharmaceutical specialities that contained povidone K 17 or povidone K 25, with samples from the original povidone batches for reference. No change in the molecular weight distribution could be determined.

Table 27. Aqueous solutions used to test for changes in the average molecular weight after sterilization or storage

Solution No.	Povidone K 12	Povidone K 17	pH (adjusted)	Sodium bisulfite addition
1	–	10%	4.0	–
2	–	10%	9.0	–
3	–	10%	9.9	0.17%
4	10%	–	6.1	–
5	20%	–	6.1	–
6	20%	–	7.0	0.4%

Table 28. The effect of sterilization (20 min at 120 –121 °C) on the relative viscosity and the average molecular weight of aqueous solutions of Kollidon® 12 PF and Kollidon® 17 PF (calculated according to Section 2.3.2.2)

Solution No.	Rel. viscosity (25 °C) Before sterilization	After sterilization	Average molecular weight ($\overline{M}v$) Before sterilization	After sterilization
1	2.10	2.09	8870	8770
2	2.08	2.08	8650	8650
3	2.11	2.07	8990	8540
4	1.65	1.67	4100	4290
5	2.67	2.70	4360	4440
6	2.65	2.62	4290	4200

Table 29. The influence of gamma radiation on the molecular weight of 10 % solutions of povidone K 17 (Kollidon® 17 PF)

Radiation dose	Molecular weight	
	Number average	Weight average
None	4 800	9 600
10 kGy	4 900	11 100
25 kGy	5 300	13 200
50 kGy	5 900	19 500

2.2.9.5
Stability of the molecular weight in liquid dosage forms after sterilization with gamma radiation

Unlike the powders, aqueous solutions of povidone are sensitive to gamma radiation. This was checked with povidone K 17 and povidone K 30. Table 29 presents the results of molecular weight measurements on povidone K 17 that was exposed, as the 10% aqueous solution, to radiation of different intensities. A clear increase in the average molecular weight and a broadening of the molecular weight distribution were found.

There are cases in which the molecular weight of the povidone grade used does not change, as it has been found that certain substances such as iodine or iodides can prevent this undesirable effect. Further, no increase in the molecular weight of a solution of povidone K 30 in a mixture of 90% polyethylene glycol and 10% water was observed after gamma irradiation.

2.3
Analytical methods for povidone

2.3.1
Qualitative and quantitative methods of determination

2.3.1.1
Identification

A series of identification reactions are described in the literature for the qualitative analysis.

The most important and clearest means of identification is provided by the infrared spectrum. It is the same for all types of povidone. Figure 24 shows the infrared spectrum of povidone K 90, and Fig. 99 shows the infrared spectra of povidone K 30 (Section 4.3.1.1). The only disadvantage of this method of identification lies in the fact that crospovidone gives the same spectrum (see Section 3.3.1.1). However, the difference can readily be determined from the solubility.

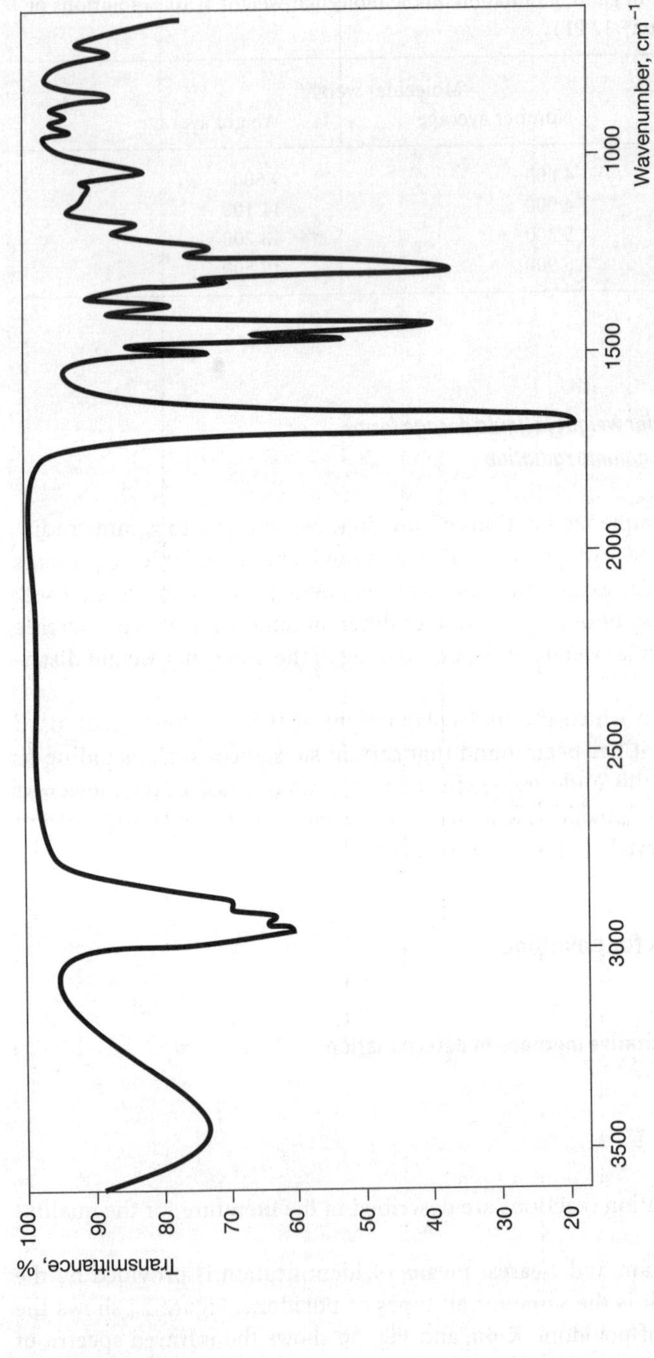

Fig. 24. Infrared spectrum of povidone K 90 recorded in potassium bromide

The following section contains the chemical identification reactions of the Pharmacopoeias for povidone. Its molecular weight determines the sensitivity of the tests.

1. An aqueous solution is mixed with a saturated solution of potassium iodide followed by 0.1 N iodine solution. A thick brown-red flocculent precipitate immediately forms.
2. 10 ml of 1 N hydrochloric acid and 2 ml of 10% potassium dichromate solution are added to 5 ml of 2% povidone solution in water. A yellow-orange precipitate forms.
3. 0.2 ml of dimethylaminobenzaldehyde reagent (0.2 g reagent + 20 ml ethanol absolute + 0.5 ml conc. hydrochloric acid decoloured with activated charcoal) and 2 ml of conc. sulfuric acid are added to 1 ml of a 2% aqueous solution of povidone. After 30 seconds, the solution is cooled. A persistent orange-pink coloration is obtained.
4. 2 ml of an aqueous solution of 75 mg cobalt nitrate and 300 mg ammonium thiocyanate is added to 5 ml of a 2% aqueous solution of povidone and the mixture acidified with 3 N hydrochloric acid. A light blue precipitate forms.

The pharmacopoeias in European countries specify identification reactions 1–3 in addition to the infrared spectrum for the identification of povidone. The U.S. Pharmacopoeia specifies reactions Nos. 1, 2, and 4 for this purpose. Further identification reactions are mentioned in Section 2.3.4.1.

The near-infrared spectrometry (NIR) can also be used for the identification of different types of povidone [619].

2.3.1.2
Quantitative methods of determination

A simple and rapid method for the quantitative determination of povidone is by photometry of the povidone-iodine complex [18, 19]:

50 ml of sample solution, which may contain up to 50 µg of povidone/ml, is mixed with 25 ml of 0.2 M citric acid solution. This is mixed with 10 ml of 0.006 N iodine solution (0.81 g of freshly sublimed iodine and 1.44 g of potassium iodide dissolved in 1000 ml of water), and after exactly 10 minutes, the absorbance of the solution is measured against a blank solution (50 ml of water + 25 ml of 0.2 M citric acid solution + 10 ml 0.006 N iodine solution) at 420 nm.

The povidone content is determined from a calibration curve, which must be plotted for each type, as their absorptivities are not the same. Fig. 25 shows the calibration curves for three different povidone grades.

A further method of determination described in the literature uses Vital Red [20, 202]. Determinations using Congo Red and by measuring the turbidity after addition of perchloric acid have also been reported.

A selective method for quantitatively determining povidone, even in traces, uses pyrolytic gas chromatography [130].

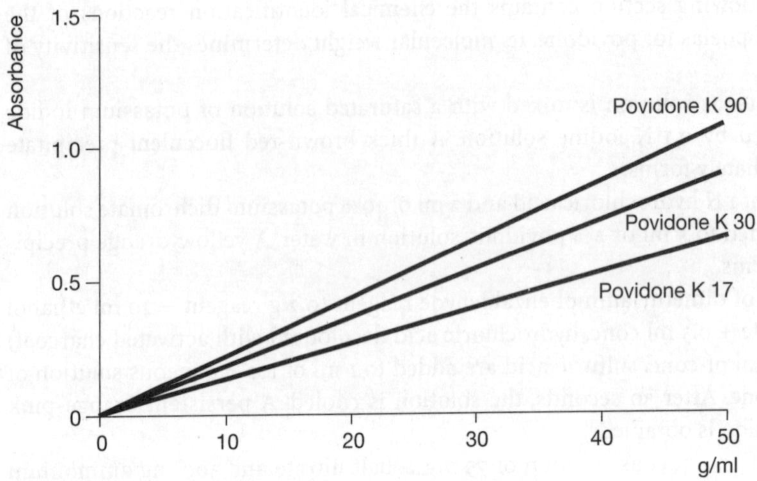

Fig. 25. Calibration curves for the photometric determination of povidone K 17, povidone K 30 and povidone K 90 with iodine

2.3.2
Methods for the determination of the K-value and molecular weight

2.3.2.1
Determination of the K-value

The significance and the official limits of the K-value have been described in Section 2.2.3.2. The value for aqueous solutions is determined according to the monographs of the Ph.Eur. and USP pharmacopoeias by methods similar to the original method [13] from the relative viscosity in water as follows.

1. Measurement of the relative viscosity, η_{rel}:
   A 5% solution is prepared, if the K-value is expected to be lower than 20, and a 1% solution, if it is expected to be over 20. The sample weights take into account the solids content of the respective povidone type, which must first be determined from the loss on drying at 105°C.
   To prepare the sample solution, a quantity of sample that has not been heated and that is exactly equivalent to 1.00 or 5.00 g of the dry product is weighed into a 100-ml volumetric flask and dissolved in a little distilled water by shaking at room temperature. The volumetric flask is then made up to the mark with water and the solution transferred to an Ubbelohde capillary viscometer (Schott & Gen, No. 1).
   It is suspended in a thermostatic bath for 30 minutes at 25 + 0.1°C, then the time taken for the solution to flow between the calibrated marks is measured several times and the average taken. To determine the relative viscosity, it is

Table 30. Calculation of the K-value from the relative viscosity

$$\log z = \frac{75 \cdot k2}{1 + 1.5 \cdot k \cdot c} + k \cdot c$$

or, according to the harmonized monograph in Ph. Eur. and USP,

$$\text{K-Value} = \frac{\sqrt{300c \cdot \log z + (c + 1.5 \cdot \log z)^2} + 1.5c \cdot \log z - c}{0.15c + 0.003c^2}$$

where

z = relative viscosity, η_{rel} of the solution at concentration c
k = K-value · 10^{-3}
c = concentration in % (w/v)

necessary to measure the flow time of water between the two marks by the same method. The Hagenbach-Couette corrections, which are enclosed with the viscometer by the manufacturer, must be subtracted from the flow times. The relative viscosity, η_{rel} is calculated as follows:

$$\eta_{rel} = \frac{\text{Flow time of the solution}}{\text{Flow time of water}}$$

2. Calculation of the K-value:
   The K-value is calculated from the relative viscosity, η_{rel} with the aid of the equation given in Table 30.

Section 2.2.3.2 contains two graphs showing the relationship between the relative viscosity and the K-value according to the above equation. However, it is preferable to use the mathematical formula as it is more accurate.

2.3.2.2
Methods for the determination of the viscosity average of the molecular weight $\bar{M}v$

In addition to the weight average of the molecular weight, which is determined by light scattering, the viscosity average, $\overline{M}v$ is becoming more and more widely used, as it is easy to determine. It can be calculated either from the K-value or from the relative viscosity via the intrinsic viscosity. Table 31 gives two equations for this purpose from the literature.

Figure 26 illustrates the relationship between the viscosity average of the molecular weight and the K-value as given by Equation 1 in Table 31.

Calculations by the two different methods in Table 31 do not always give the same results. As can be seen from Fig. 27, this is particularly evident at higher K-

Table 31. Equations for the calculation of the viscosity average of the molecular weight, $\bar{M}v$ of povidone

1. Calculation of Mv from the K-value [212]

$$\bar{M}v = 22.22\ (K + 0.075\ K^2)^{1.65}$$

2. Calculation of $\bar{M}v$ from the relative viscosity via the intrinsic viscosity

A. Intrinsic viscosity [16]:

$$[\eta] = \frac{\eta_{rel} - 1}{c + 0.28\ c\ (\eta_{rel} - 1)}$$

B. Viscosity average [15]:

$$\bar{M}v = 8.04 \cdot 10^5\ [\eta]^{1.82}$$

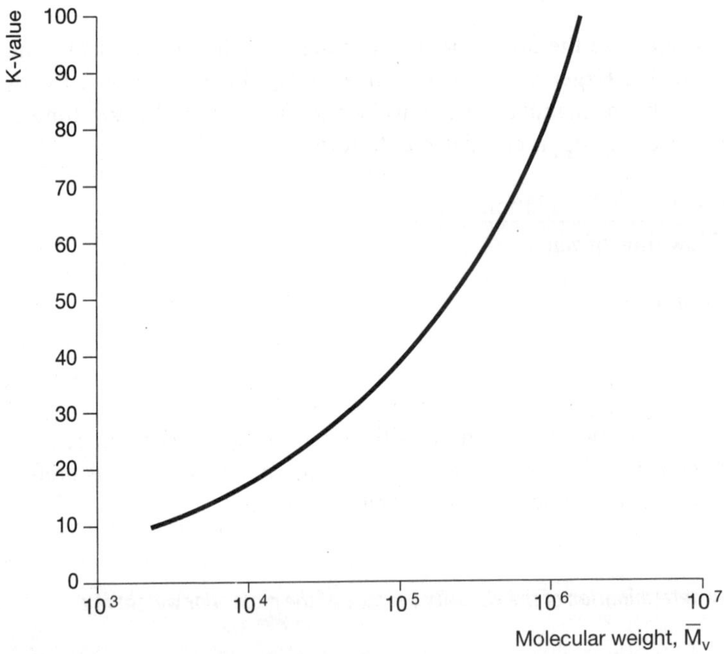

Fig. 26. Relationship between the K-value and the viscosity average of the molecular weight, Mv, calculated with equation 1 in Table 31

values. The viscosity average of the molecular weight calculated from the K-value with Equation 1 is lower than that calculated with the other equation. The same relative viscosities were taken for the calculation of both the K-value and the intrinsic viscosity.

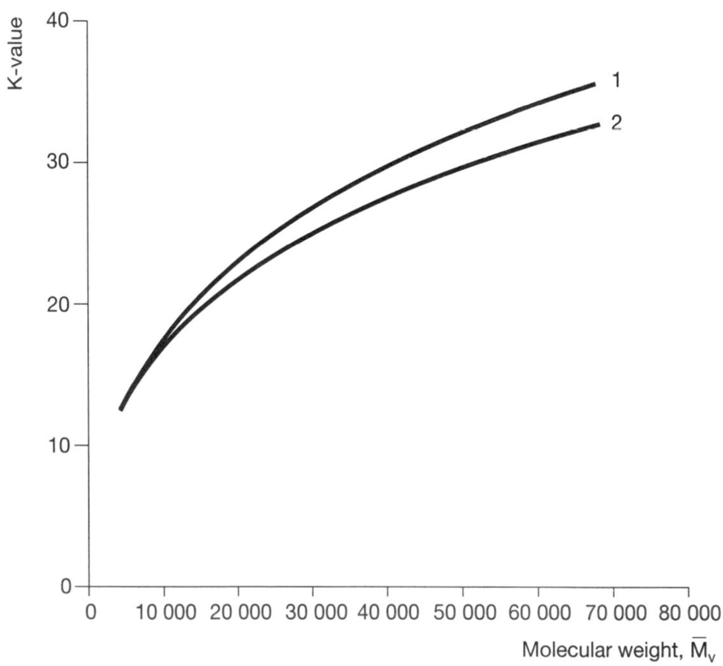

Fig. 27. Relationship between K-values from 12 to 33 and the viscosity average of the molecular weight, calculated by different methods
1: Equation 1 from Table 31; 2: Equations 2 A + B from Table 31

2.3.3
Methods for the determination of purity

2.3.3.1
Pharmacopoeia methods

Methods for determining the purity of povidone are described in detail in the European, U.S. and Japanese pharmacopoeias. They cover all the parameters listed in Table 32.

Some of the former pharmacopoeial methods are not always entirely relevant. This applies particularly to the titration tests of vinylpyrrolidone or aldehydes, as the methods are not specific and inaccurate, and therefore no longer do justice to the purity of povidone availabe today. For this reason, the harmonized monograph "Povidone" introduced an HPLC method for vinylpyrrolidone and an enzymatic test for acetaldehyde.

Table 32. Purity test methods for povidone given in pharmacopoeias

Colour and clarity of solution
Acetaldehyde
pH
Vinylpyrrolidone (= Impurity A)
2-Pyrrolidone (= Impurity B)
Hydrazine
Peroxides
Water
Sulphated ash =residue on ignition
Heavy metals
Residual solvents (Formic acid or 2-propanol)
Organic volatile impurities
Nitrogen
Microbial status
Endotoxins

2.3.3.2
HPLC method for the determination of free N-vinylpyrrolidone, 2-pyrrolidone and vinyl acetate in povidone and copovidone

Principle:
A sample of povidone or copovidone is analyzed after dissolution in a water/ methanol mixture using HPLC reverse phase chromatography (gradient run). The polymeric material is kept away from the chromatographic system using a precolumn and switching technique.

The determination limits are 2 mg/kg N-vinylpyrrolidone, 200 mg/kg 2-pyrrolidone and 10 mg/kg vinyl acetate.

Sample preparation:
Weight about 250 mg of povidone or copovidone in a 10 ml volumetric flask, add 1 ml of methanol and apply ultrasonic action until complete dissolution is achieved. Fill up to volume with water. If the sample of povidone K90 is not dissolved completely in methanol stirr after filling up to volume with water until the complete dissolution. Aliquotes of this sample solution are used for injection after filtration.

For samples of povidone containing more than 1.5 g/100 g 2-pyrrolidone (e.g. povidone K 25 and K 30), the sample weight has to be reduced if the linear range of calibration is exceeded.

Calibration solutions:
Dissolve reference substances (50 mg of N-vinylpyrrolidone, about 300 mg of 2-pyrrolidone and 50 mg of vinyl acetate in the case of copovidone) in methanol and dilute with the same solvent. Further dilutions are done with eluent A.

At least two sample weights of each reference substance and at least four concentrations derived thereof are used for the calibration curve.

The concentrations have to be selected in such a way that the concentration of the individual analyte in the sample is included.

Concerning the determination of 2-pyrrolidone, calibration up to about 1.5 g per 100 g of sample usually is linear.

When starting the analysis, precolumn and separation column are in series. After 2.5 min (depending on the separation characteristics of the precolumn) column switching is applied in such way that the eluent is guided directly onto the separation column avoiding the precolumn. The precolumn is simultaneously flushed backwards in order to eliminate the polymer components. After 40 min the system is set back for the next injection (Table 34, Fig. 28).

Calculation of the calibration factor:

$$KF = \frac{FK}{\beta(K)} \quad \frac{mV\,s\;10\;ml}{mg}$$

KF = Calibration factor
FK = Peak area of the reference substance 2-pyrrolidone resp. N-vinyl pyrrolidone resp. vinyl acetate
ß(K) = Calculated concentration of the reference substance

Table 33. Chromatographic conditions

• Column:	250 x 4 mm packed with Aquasil® C18, 5 µm (ThermoHypersil)		
• Precolumn:	30 x 4 mm packed with Nucleosil® 120-5 C18 (Macherey & Nagel)		
• Mobile phases:	Eluent A: water + acetonitrile + methanol (90+5+5, v/v/v)		
	Eluent B: water + acetonitrile + methanol (50+45+5, v/v/v)		
• Gradient run:	t (min)	% Eluent A	% Eluent B
	0	100	0
	26	80	20
	27	0	100
	38	100	0
• Flow rate:	1.0 ml/min		
• Injection volume:	10 µl		
• Detection:	UV (205 nm and 233 nm)		
• Column temperature:	30°C		
• Rf value of 2-pyrrolidone:	about 6 min		
• Rf value of vinyl acetate:	about 17 min		
• Rf value of N-vinylpyrrolidone:	about 21 min		

Table 34. Chromatographic run scheme:

T (min)	Action/State of system
0	Eluent A
0,1	Detector wave length 205 nm
0,2	Base line reset
2.5	Column switching
19.6	Detector wave length 233 nm
19.7	Base line reset
26.0	Eluent B 20 %
27.0	Eluent B 100 %
38.0	Eluent A
40.0	Column switching
53.0	Next injection

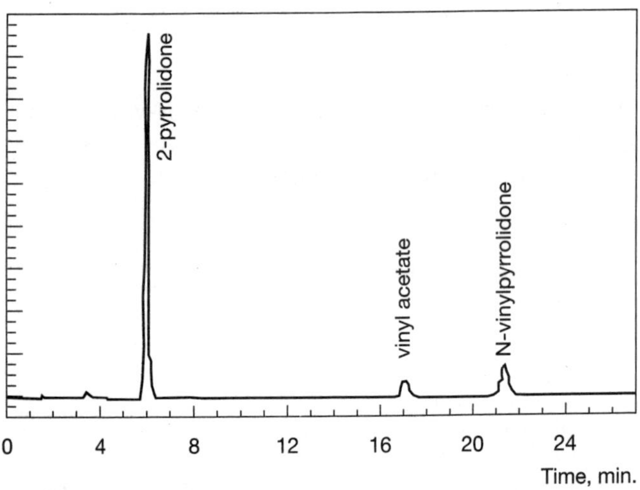

Fig. 28. Typical chromatogram of the three reference substances

Calculation of 2-pyrrolidone resp. N-vinylpyrrolidone resp. vinyl acetate in the sample:

$$w(P) = \frac{FP}{KF \cdot \beta[P]} \times 100$$

$w(P)$ = Mass fraction of 2-pyrrolidone resp. N-vinylpyrrolidone resp. vinyl acetate in the sample [g/100 g]

KF = Calibration factor

FP = Peak area of 2-pyrrolidone resp. N-vinylpyrrolidone resp. vinyl acetate in the sample chromatogram [mV s]

ß(P) = calculated concentration of the sample solution [mg/10 ml]

Validation

Linearity:

The calibration curves given in Fig. 29, 30 and 31 were obtained with the reference substances 2-pyrrolidone, N-vinylpyrrolidone and vinyl acetate.

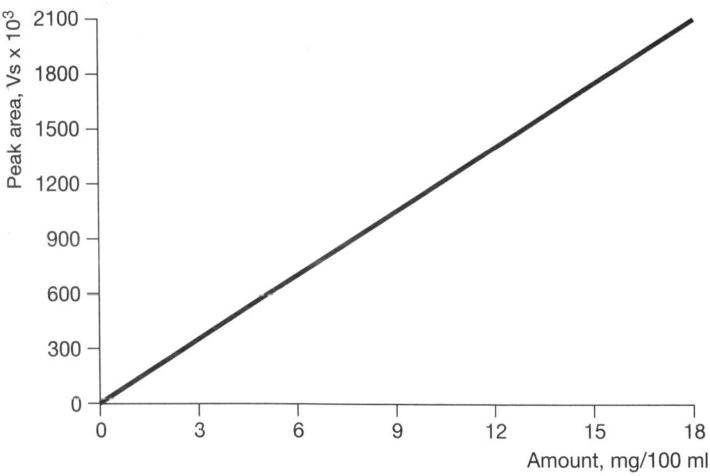

Fig. 29. Calibration curve of 2-pyrrolidone

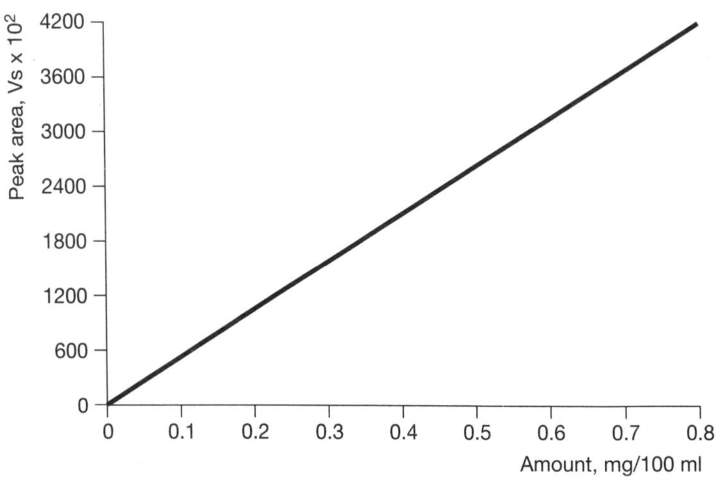

Fig. 30. Calibration curve of N-vinylpyrrolidone

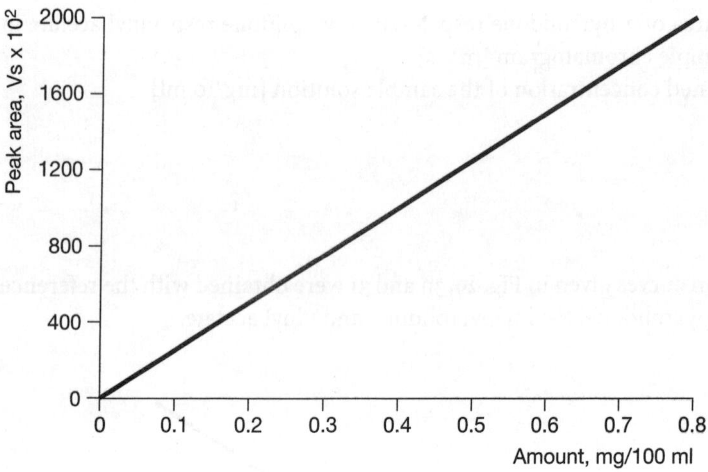

Fig. 31. Calibration curve of vinyl acetate

Reproducibility:

The content of the 2-pyrrolidone and N-vinylpyrrolidone was determined six times on povidone K 30 (Kollidon® 30, batch 13128775L0) (Table 35).

The content of the 2-pyrrolidone and N-vinylpyrrolidone was determined six times on povidone K 17 (Kollidon® 17PF, batch 80472716K0) (Table 36).

The content of the 2-pyrrolidone, N-vinylpyrrolidone and vinyl acetate was determined six times on copovidone (Kollidon® VA64, batch 19265124U0) (Table 37).

Table 35. Reproducibility on povidone K 30

	2-Pyrrolidone [g/100 g]	N-Vinylpyrrolidone [mg/kg]
1. Measurement	1.174	<2
2. Measurement	1.191	<2
3. Measurement	1.178	<2
4. Measurement	1.170	<2
5. Measurement	1.160	<2
6. Measurement	1.149	<2
Average	*1.17*	<2
Rel. standard deviation	*1 %*	

Table 36. Reproducibility on povidone K 17

	2-Pyrrolidone [g/100 g]	N-Vinylpyrrolidone [mg/kg]
1. Measurement	537	<2
2. Measurement	533	<2
3. Measurement	536	<2
4. Measurement	535	<2
5. Measurement	539	<2
6. Measurement	533	<2
Average	*536*	*<2*
Rel. standard deviation	*<1 %*	

Table 37. Reproducibility on copovidone

	2-Pyrrolidone [mg/kg]	N-Vinylpyrrolidone [mg/kg]	Vinyl acetate [mg/kg]
1. Measurement	441	8.9	<10
2. Measurement	439	8.6	<10
3. Measurement	440	8.7	<10
4. Measurement	440	8.8	<10
5. Measurement	442	8.7	<10
6. Measurement	442	8.8	<10
Average	*441*	*8.7*	*<10*
Rel. standard deviation	*<1 %*	*1 %*	

Recovery

The content of 2-pyrrolidone and N-vinylpyrrolidone was determined in povidone before and after addition of two different amounts of the reference substances (Table 38).

The content of 2-pyrrolidone, N-vinylpyrrolidone and vinyl acetate was determined in copovidone before and after addition of different amounts of the reference substances (Table 39).

Table 38. Recovery in povidone K30

	Initial value [mg/kg]	Added amount [mg/kg]	Theoretical content [mg/kg]	Found content [mg/kg]	Recovery rate [mg/kg]
2-Pyrrolidone	11 700	223	11 923	11 860	71 %
	11 700	412	12 112	12 120	101 %
N-Vinylpyrro-lidone	1.5	10.9	12.4	9.0	69 %
	1.5	20.2	21.7	23.6	109 %

Table 39. Recovery in copovidone:

	Initial value [mg/kg]	Added amount [mg/kg]	Theoretical content [mg/kg]	Found content [mg/kg]	Recovery rate [mg/kg]
2-Pyrrolidone	441	79	520	520	100 %
	441	325	766	777	103 %
N-Vinylpyrro-lidone	8.7	3.9	12.6	12.4	94 %
	8.7	15.9	24.6	24.5	99 %
Vinyl acetate	<10	16.0	16.0	16.1	100 %
		26.9	26.9	26.0	97 %
		60.1	60.1	57.0	95 %

Comparison with the methods of the povidone monograph in Ph.Eur. 5

The batches of povidone and of copovidone mentioned in the section Reproducibility were tested in parallel with this HPLC method and the Ph.Eur. methods for 2-pyrrolidone and N-vinylpyrrolidone. Table 40 illustrates the resultsobtained with the Ph.Eur. methods. The results are comparable with the results mentioned under Reproducibility (Tables 35 to 37) (Table 41, 42).

Table 40. Results of the Ph.Eur. methods on povidone K 30

	2-Pyrrolidone [g/100 g]	N-Vinylpyrrolidone [mg/kg]
1. Measurement	1.27	1.4
2. Measurement	1.27	1.4
3. Measurement	1.28	1.3
4. Measurement	1.27	1.4
5. Measurement	1.28	1.3
6. Measurement	1.26	1.3
Average	*1.27*	*1.3*
Rel. standard deviation	*<1 %*	*2 %*

Table 41. Results of the Ph.Eur. methods on povidone K 17

	2-Pyrrolidone [mg/kg]	N-Vinylpyrrolidone [mg/kg]
1. Measurement	520	<1
2. Measurement	505	<1
3. Measurement	480	<1
4. Measurement	446	<1
5. Measurement	437	<1
6. Measurement	463	<1
Average	*475*	*<1*
Rel. standard deviation	*6 %*	

Table 42. Results of the Ph.Eur. methods on copovidone

	2-Pyrrolidone [mg/kg]	N-Vinylpyrrolidone [mg/kg]
1. Measurement	368	9.2
2. Measurement	353	9.1
3. Measurement	359	9.1
4. Measurement	344	8.9
5. Measurement	365	9.0
6. Measurement	368	9.0
Average	*360*	*9.1*
Rel. standard deviation	*2.4 %*	*1 %*

2.3.3.3
Enzymatic determination of acetaldehyde

As the titration method for the determination of acetaldehyde is very unspecific and measures more than just aldehydes or acetaldehyde, the following specific enzymatic method is recommended. It was introduced in the harmonized monograph of povidone in Ph.Eur., USP and JP.

Principle:
Acetaldehyde is stoichiometrically oxidized to acetic acid by nicotinamide-adenine dinucleotide (NAD) in the presence of aldehyde dehydrogenase. This method measures the sum of free and bound acetaldehyde.

$$\text{Acetaldehyde} + NAD^+ + H_2O \xrightarrow{\text{Al-DH}} \text{Acetic acid} + NADH + H^+$$

Reagent solutions:
I. Buffer (potassium dihydrogen phosphate, 0.05 mol/l, pH 9.0): Dissolve 1.74 g of KH_2PO_4 in about 80 ml water, adjust to pH 9.0 with 1 mol/l potassium hydroxyde and make up to 100 ml with water. The solution is stable for two months at 4 °C.
II. Nicotinamide-adenine dinucleotide solution, NAD: Dissolve 40 mg of NAD (e.g. Boehringer Mannheim Order No. 127329) in 10 ml of water. The solution is stable for four weeks at 4 °C.
III. Aldehyde dehydrogenase, Al-DH (7 U/ml): Dissolve 7 units of aldehyde dehydrogenase lyophilisate (e.g. Boehringer Mannheim Order No. 171832) in 1.0 ml of water. The solution is stable for eight hours at 4 °C or for two days when frozen.

Sample solution:
Weigh 200–500 mg of the povidone sample (W, mg), accurate to 0.2 mg, into a 10-ml volumetric flask, dissolve in buffer (I) and make up to the mark with buffer (I). Heat the closed flask for 60 minutes at 60 °C, then cool to room temperature.

Procedure:
Mix 0.2 ml of NAD solution (II) with 3 ml of the sample solution in a 1-cm photometric cell and measure the absorbance at 340 nm against water (A_{0S}). Add 0.05 ml of Al-DH solution (III), mix and, after 5 min measure the absorbance at 340 mm against water again (A_{1S}).

Conduct a blank determination using 3 ml of buffer (I) instead of the sample solution (A_{0B} and A_{1B}).

Calculation:

$$\text{ppm acetaldehyde} = \frac{75\,750}{W} \cdot [(A_{1S} - A_{0S}) - (A_{1B} - A_{0B})]$$

Validation

Linearity:
Measurements with pure acetaldehyde with a concentration of 5–55 µg/10 ml demonstrate the linearity of the method with a correlation coefficient of 0.99998.

Reproducibility:
The acetaldehyde content of a sample of povidone K 30 was determined 6 times. The values found, the average and the relative standard deviation are given in Table 43.

Recovery rate:
To a sample of povidone (Kollidon® 30 batch 822) different amounts of acetaldehyde-ammonia trimer (=Hexahydro 2.4.6-trimethyl 1.3.5 triazine, $C_6H_{15}N_3 \cdot 3H_2O$, CAS number 76231-37-3, available at Fluka/Sigma Aldrich) were added and determined enzymatically. The acetaldehyde in this Kollidon® batch was 45 mg/kg before the addition (Table 44).

Table 43. Acetaldehyde content of a povidone K 30 sample (Kollidon® 30)

Determination No.	Acetaldehyde [mg/kg]
1	102.0
2	103.3
3	102.6
4	103.6
5	100.4
Average	102.4
s_{rel}	1.1%

Table 44. Recovery on povidone K 30

Added acetaldehyde – ammonia trimer (calculated as acetaldehyde) [mg/kg]	Theoretical content of acetaldehyde [mg/kg]	Found acetaldehyde [mg/kg]	Recovery rate [%]
46 mg/kg	91	91	100
58 mg/kg	103	102	98
77 mg/kg	122	120	97
92 mg/kg	137	134	97
111 mg/kg	161	158	97

Notes:
Because of the volatility of acetaldehyde, all flasks and cells must be well sealed during the determination.

Acetaldehyde for calibration purposes must be distilled before use.

If the sample solution is not heated to 60 °C, only the free acetaldehyde is determined and proper validation is not possible.

2.3.3.4
Enzymatic determination of formic acid

Principle:
Formic acid is oxidized in the presence of formate dehydrogenase (FDH) by nicotinamide-adenine dinucleotide (NAD) quantitatively to bicarbonate.

The amount of NADH formed during this reaction is stoichiometric with the amount of formic acid. The increase in NADH is measured by means of its absorbance at 340 nm.

Reagents:
Test combination of Boehringer/Mannheim (Germany, Catalogue No. 979 732):
- Bottle 1: 22 ml of potassium phosphate buffer pH 7.5, stabilizer.
- Bottle 2: 420 mg NAD lithium salt, lyophilisate.
- Bottle 3: 200 mg formate dehydrogenase (FDH), lyophilisate, 80 U.

Preparation of the reagent solutions:
1. Dissolve the content of bottle 2 with the content of bottle 1 (= NAD solution 2, stable for 2 weeks at 4 °C, to use at 20–25 °C)
2. Dissolve the content of bottle 3 with 1.2 ml of water (= FDH enzyme solution 3, stable for 20 days at 4 °C).

Sample solution:
Weight accurately approx. 3 g of povidone into a volumetric flask. Fill up with 60–70 ml of water and dissolve the sample completely. Fill up to the mark with water and shake.

Measurement:
In two glass cuvettes with stopper pipette the following amounts

	blank	sample
NAD solution 2	1.00 ml	1.00 ml
Water	2.00 ml	1.90 ml
Sample solution	–	0.10 ml

Shake the cuvettes and after 5 min measure against air the absorbances at 340 nm of the sample cuvette (Eos) and of the blank (Eob). Now start the enzyme reaction by adding 0.05 ml of the FDH enzyme solution 3 into both cuvettes. Wait for 20 min at 20–25 °C and measure the absorbances again of the blank (E1b) and the sample (E1s) against air.

Calculation:

$$E = (E1_s - E0_s) - (E1_b - E0_b)$$

$$C[\%] = \frac{E \cdot 2.229}{\text{Sample [g]}}$$

Validation

Linearity:
The calibration curve of formic acid was plotted from 6 points covering a concentration range of 10–220 µg/ml to check their linearity (Table 45).

Reproducibility:
The formic acid content of povidone (batch 719 of Kollidon® 30) was determined in 5 times (Table 46).

Table 45. Calibration results with formic acid

Concentration of formic acid [µg/ml]	Absorbance 340 nm
10.9	0.049
20.3	0.091
42.1	0.189
107.7	0.483
172.3	0.773
219.8	0.960

Table 46. Recovery of formic acid in povidone K 30

Measurement	Formic acid (%)
1.	0.2697
2.	0.2683
3.	0.2674
4.	0.2647
5.	0.2666
Average	0.2673
Standard deviation	17

Table 47. Recovery of formic acid in povidone K 30

Formic acid added [mg]	Formic acid found [mg]	Recovery rate [%]
4.38	4.06	93
6.03	5.68	94
8.04	7.66	95
10.95	10.74	98

Recovery rate:
To the same batch 719 of povidone K 30 different known amounts of formic acid were added and determined (Table 47).

2.3.3.5
GC Determination of 2-propanol (isopropanol) in low-molecular povidone and in copovidone

Principle:
The determination of 2-propanol can be done by the following modified gaschromatographic method given in ISO 13741-1.

Internal standard solution. Weight about 250 mg of propionitrile, dissolve it in water and dilute to 1000 ml with the same solvent.

Test solution. Weight about 10 g of the povidone (copovidone) sample and dissolve in 30 g of the internal standard solution (Table 48).

Table 48. Modified chromatographic conditions

• Column:	DB-wax 30 m x 0.25 mm, film 1 µm
• Carrier gas:	Nitrogen
• Flow rate of carrier gas:	1 ml/min
• Split:	1 : 30
• Detector:	FID
• Injection volume:	1 µl
• Temperature injection block:	200°C
• Temperature detector:	200°C
• Temperature program, column:	a. 3 min at 50°C b. Heating from 50° to 200°C with 20°C/min c. 200°C during 37.5 min
• Rf value of propionitrile	about 6.6
• Rf value of 2-propanol	about 4.4

2.3.3.6
Determination of nitrogen in povidone and crospovidone

As the description of the nitrogen determination in the povidone (and crospovidone) monographs included in Ph.Eur. 5 and in USP26 is not exact enough to obtain always a complete degradation of the polyvinylpyrrolidone polymer a modified Ph.Eur. method is given here:

Place 450.0 mg of the substance to be examined (m mg) in a combustion flask, add 10 g of a mixture of 48.9 g of *dipotassium sulphate R, 48.8 g disodium sulphate R* and 0.3 g of *copper sulphate R,* and 3 glass beads. Wash any adhering particles from the neck into the flask with a small quantity of *sulphuric acid R.* Add in total 20 ml of sulphuric acid R, allowing it to run down the sides of the flask, and mix the contents by rotation. Close the mouth of the flask loosely, for example by means of a glass bulb with a short stem, to avoid excessive loss of sulphuric acid. Heat gradually at first,then increase the temperature until there is vigorous boiling with condensation of sulphuric acid in the neck of the flask; precautions are to be taken to prevent the upper part of the flask from becoming overheated. Continue the heating for 60 minutes until a completely clear greenish solution is obtained. Cool, cautiously add to the mixture 35 ml of water R, and after 10 seconds add 65 ml of *strong sodium hydroxide solution R,* cool again and place in a steam-distillation apparatus. Distill immediately by passing steam through the mixture. Collect about 150 ml of distillate in a mixture of 100 ml of a 40 g/l solution of boric acid R and 3 drops of *bromcresol green-methyl red solution R* and 100 ml of *water R* to cover the tip of the condenser. Towards the end of the distillation lower the receiver so that the tip of the condenser is above the surface of the acid solution and rinse the end part of the condenser with a small quantity of water R. Titrate the distillate with *0.25 M sulphuric acid* until the colour of the solution changes from green through pale greyish-blue to pale greyish-red-purple ($n_1$ml of *0.25 M sulphuric acid).*

Repeat the test using about 450.0 mg of glucose R in place of the substance to be examined ($n_2$ml of *0.25 M sulphuric acid*).

$$\text{nitrogen (per cent)} = \frac{700.4\ (n_1 - n_2)}{\text{m}\ (100 - \text{d})} \times 100$$

d = loss on drying, %

2.3.3.7
GC Determination of (hydroxy-methyl)-butylpyrrolidone (= "2-propanol-vinylpyrrolidone adduct") in low-molecular povidone

As the low-molecular povidone types are polymerized in 2-propanol instead of water small amounts of the radical adduct of 2-propanol to the monomer N-vinylpyrrolidone can be formed (Fig. 32).

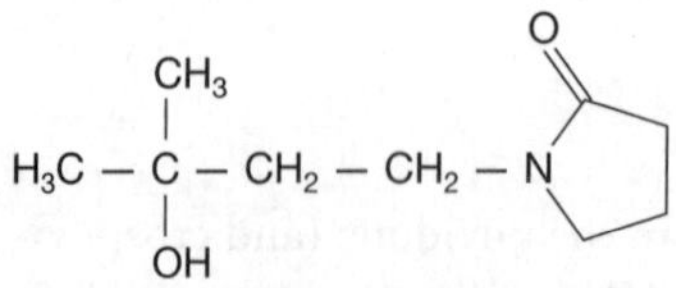

Fig. 32. (3'-Hydroxy,3'-methyl)-N-butylpyrrolidin-2-one ("HMBP")

The detection limit of this gaschromatographic method is about 100 mg/kg.
Preparation of solutions:
Internal standard solution Weight about 0.125 g of *benzonitrile* and dissolve it in *anhydrous ethanol* (Ph.Eur.) and dilute to 100 ml with the same solvent. Ditute 10 ml of this solution to 250 ml with *anhydrous ethanol* (= 0.05 mg/ml).

Reference solution. Weight about 0.1 g of *(3'-Hydroxy,3'-methyl)-N-butyl-pyrrolidin-2-one (HMBP),* dissolve in *anhydrous ethanol* and dilute to 100 ml with the same solvent (= 1 mg/ml).

Calibration solutions. For the determination of the calibration factor prepare at least three calibration solutions by mixing 20 ml of the *internal standard solution* with different amounts between 1 and 10 ml of the *reference* solution and by diluting to 50 ml with *anhydrous ethanol.*

Test solution. Weight about 0.2 g of the povidone sample, dissolve in 5 ml of the internal standard solution and dilute to 25 ml with anhydrous ethanol (Table 49).

Table 49. Chromatographic conditions

• Column:	DB-wax 30 m x 0.25 mm, film 0.5 µm (J&W Scientific)
• Carrier gas:	Helium, 1 bar
• Flow rate of carrier gas:	1 ml/min
• Split:	1 : 60
• Nitrogen detector	
• Injection volume:	1 µl
• Temperature injection block:	240°C
• Temperature detector:	260°C
• Temperature program, column:	a. Heating from 180° to 240°C with 4°C/min b. 240°C during 7.5 min c. Cooling from 240° to 180°C with 8–9°C/min

Calculation of the calibration factor:
Calculate the calibration factor F of each calibration solution and the average of the obtained factors (= F_{av}).

$$F = \frac{A_s \times C_r}{A_r \times C_s}$$

A_s = peak aerea of the internal standard benzonitrile (mV · s)
A_r = peak aerea of the reference substance (mV · s)
C_s = concentration of the internal standard in the calibration solution (µg/ml)
C_r = concentration of the reference substance in the calibration solution (µg/ml)

Calculation of the content of the 2-propanol-vinylpyrrolidone adduct HMBP in the sample (Fig. 33):

$$\text{Content of HMBP (ppm)} = \frac{C_{st} \times 5}{W} \times \frac{F_{av} \times A_a \times 1000}{A_{st}}$$

A_{st} = peak aerea of the internal standard benzonitrile (mV · s)
A_a = peak aerea of the 2-propanol-vinylpyrrolidone adduct HMBP (mV · s)
C_{st} = concentration of benzonitril in the internal standard solution (mg/ml)
F_{av} = average calibration factor
W = Weight of the sample of povidone (g)

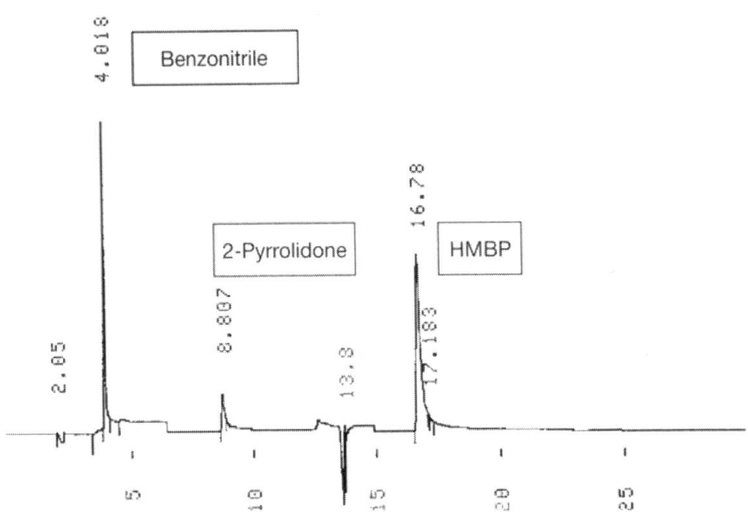

Fig. 33. Typical GC chromatogram of povidone K 17 (Kollidon® 17PF)

Validation

Linearity:
The calibration curve was plotted from five different points covering a concentration range of 9 to 200 µg HMBP/ml (Fig. 34).

Recovery:
The content of the 2-propanol-vinylpyrrolidone adduct (HMBP) was determined twice on both low-molecular povidones before and after addition of different amounts of HMBP. Table 50 shows the results.

Reproducibility:
The content of the 2-propanol-vinylpyrrolidone adduct (HMBP) was determined five times on batch 932 of Kollidon® 17PF (Table 51).

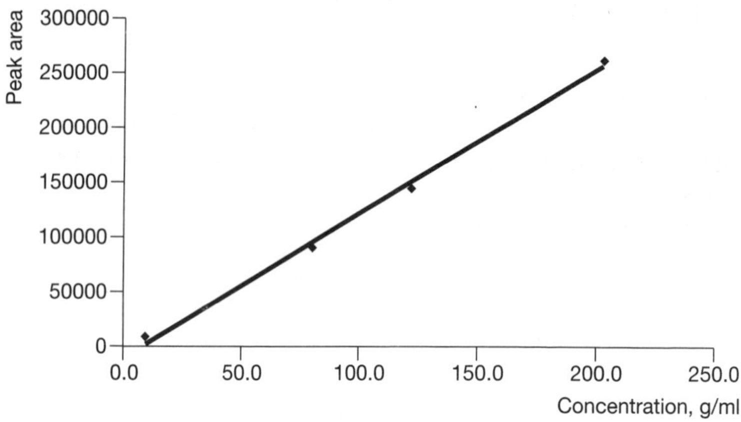

Fig. 34. Calibration curve of HMBP

Table 50. Recovery of added HMBP in povidone K 12 and povidone K 17

	Initial value [mg/kg]	Added amount [mg/kg]	Theoretical content [mg/kg]	Found content [mg/kg]	Recovery rate [%]
Kollidon® 12PF, batch 378	11 100	10 400	21 500	23 290	108
Kollidon® 12PF, batch 378	11 100	14 690	25 790	29 760	115
Kollidon® 17PF, batch 923	3 280	4 880	8 160	8 490	104
Kollidon® 17PF, batch 923	3 280	13 220	16 500	17 895	108

Table 51. Reproducibility on povidone K 17

	HMBP found
1. Measurement	3 837 ppm
2. Measurement	3 824 ppm
3. Measurement	3 594 ppm
4. Measurement	3 644 ppm
5. Measurement	3 671 ppm
Average	3714 ppm
Standard deviation	90

2.3.4 Determination of povidone in preparations

2.3.4.1 *Qualitative determination*

The various means of detecting povidone in preparations have been described in detail in the literature [17, 18]. Not all the detection reactions listed in Table 52 (see also Section 2.3.1.1) are suitable for every pharmaceutical preparation. The best method can only be determined by trial with the preparation involved.

The separation scheme shown in Fig. 35 can be used for the detection of povidone in solid dosage forms, e.g. tablets, granules, capsules and coated tablets.

The detection and differentiation of povidone and copovidone obtained in Fraction A I in Fig. 35 is best carried out by thin layer chromatography on silica gel or paper. A suitable eluent is a mixture of 6 parts n-propanol and 4 parts 2N ammonia solution by volume, which gives the Rf values shown in Table 53. The chromatogram is then sprayed with Lugol's solution.

Electrophoresis can also be used to detect povidone in the presence of copovidone [17].

Povidone can be detected in tissue with the aid of chlorazol or Congo Red [143, 144].

Table 52. Detection reactions for povidone [18]

Reagent	Reaction
10% aqueous barium chloride solution + 1 N hydrochloric acid + 5% aqueous silicotungstic acid solution	White precipitate
10% aqueous barium chloride solution + 1 N hydrochloric acid + 5% aqueous phosphotungstic acid solution	Yellow precipitate
10% potassium dichromate solution + 1 N hydrochloric acid	Orange-yellow precipitate
Saturated aqueous potassium bromide solution + bromine water	Orange-yellow precipitate
Saturated aqueous potassium iodide solution + 0.1 N iodine solution	Brown-red precipitate
Dragendorff's reagent + 1 N hydrochloric acid	Brown-red precipitate
Neßler's Reagent	Yellow-white precipitate
Saturated aqueous potassium ferrocyanide solution + 6 N hydrochloric acid	White precipitate
Saturated aqueous potassium ferricyanide solution + 6 N hydrochloric acid	Yellow precipitate
Aqueous ammonium cobalt rhodanide solution + 6 N hydrochloric acid	Blue precipitate
Concentrated aqueous phenol solution	White precipitate

Table 53. Rf values for povidone and copovidone separated by thin layer and paper chromatography using propanol + ammonia solution (6 + 4) as eluent [17]

Substance	Rf values	
	Silica gel plate	FP 3 paper
Povidone	0.59–0.64	0.33–0.66
Copovidone	0.64–0.75	0.72–1.00

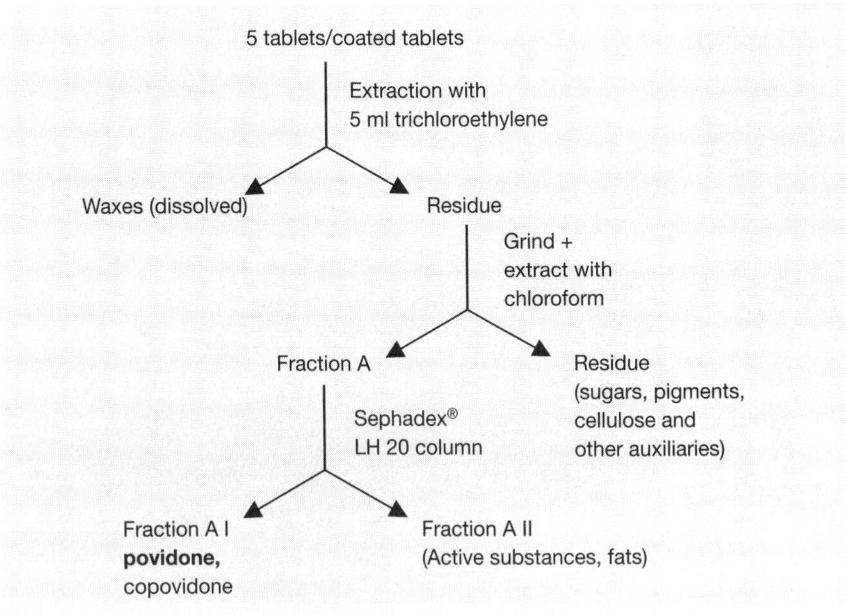

Fig. 35. Separation scheme for the isolation of povidone in solid dosage forms [17]

2.3.4.2
Quantitative determination in preparations

The most versatile method for quantitatively determining povidone is probably the photometric measurement of the povidone-iodine complex described in Section 2.3.1.2. It has been successfully tested on samples that also contained a series of auxiliaries and drugs [18].

In these tests, aqueous solutions containing 50, 100 and 200 µg of povidone and 20 times the quantity of the tablet ingredients listed below were prepared, and their povidone content determined.

The following tablet ingredients were incorporated:

Acetylsalicylic acid
Ascorbic acid
Bromoisovalerylurea
Caffeine
Diphenhydramine hydrochloride
Ephedrine hydrochloride
Ethylpapaverine
Glucose
Lactose
Lidocaine
Meprobamate
Monophenylbutazone
Acetphenetidine
Phenobarbital
Phenyldimethylpyrazolone
Salicylamide
Sodium salicylate
Starch
Tartaric acid
Thiamine hydrochloride

Table 54. Photometric determination of povidone K 25 in the presence of different compounds [18]

Povidone K 25 added, μg	μg of povidone, recovered in the presence of 20 times the quantity of:											
	Lactose	Glucose	Tartaric acid	Acetyl-salicylic acid	Thiamine hydro-chloride	Brom-isoval	Caffeine	Ephedrine hydro-chloride	Lidocaine	Meproba-mate	Pheno-barbital	Salicyl-amide
50	48	49	47	48	47	49	50	50	46	48	46	50
100	100	99	99	99	99	99	102	99	97	99	97	100
200	199	200	201	198	203	197	203	202	195	200	200	204

Table 55. Photometric determination of povidone K 25 by the modified general method [18].

Povidone added, μg	μg of povidone recovered in the presence of 20 times the quantity of: Phenyldimethylpyrazolone	Diphenhydramine hydrochloride	Ethylpapaverine	Monophenylbutazone	Ascorbic acid	Starch
50	47	52	51	52	49	48
100	96	100	100	101	97	96
200	195	200	198	200	196	196

Table 54 shows that povidone can be determined with sufficient accuracy in the presence of 12 of the compounds listed above.

Phenyldimethylpyrazolone, diphenhydramine, ethylpapaverine, monophenylbutazone, ascorbic acid and starch react with iodine. The general method, in which iodine is used as a reagent, cannot be used directly if these substances are present. However, it is possible to pretreat the samples to enable povidone to be determined in solutions that contain these substances. Phenyldimethylpyrazolone, diphenhydramine hydrochloride, ethyl papaverine and monophenylbutazone can be extracted by shaking the aqueous solution with a suitable organic solvent in a separating funnel.

The povidone remains in the aqueous phase and can then be determined by the general method. Ethyl papaverine and diphenhydramine hydrochloride can be extracted with cyclohexanol from the alkaline aqueous solution; monophenylbutazone can be extracted from neutral aqueous solutions with the same solvent. Phenyldimethylpyrazolone can be removed from alkaline aqueous solutions by extraction with chloroform. Unlike povidone, starch is insoluble in methanol. The evaporation residue of a solution containing starch and povidone is therefore treated with methanol; povidone can then be determined by the general method in the methanolic solution after filtration.

If ascorbic acid is present, this is stoichiometrically oxidized to dehydroascorbic acid, which does not interfere with the determination, by titration with iodine solution.

Table 55 shows the results of analyses of solutions containing the interfering substances by the general method with the modification described above.

Methods for the determination of povidone in contact lens fluids with the aid of Congo Red [142] as well as a fluorimetric method that uses anilinenaphthaline sulfonate [111, 181] are described in the literature.

A UV-spectrophotometric determination of more than 20% of povidone K 30 in mixtures with active ingredients was developed by multicomponent analysis [618].

2.4 Applications of povidone

2.4.1 General properties

Povidone possess a number of very useful properties for which they are widely used in pharmaceuticals.

Because of these properties, the products can perform different functions in different dosage forms (Table 56).

The excellent *solubility* in water and in other solvents used in pharmaceutical production (Section 2.2.2) is an advantage in almost all dosage forms, e.g. in wet granulation in tablet production, in oral solutions, syrups and drops, in injectables and topical solutions and in film coatings on tablets.

The *adhesive and binding power* is particularly important in tabletting (wet granulation, dry granulation, direct compression). This property is also useful in film coatings and adhesive gels.

The *film-forming properties* are used in the film-coating of tablets, in transdermal systems and in medicinal sprays.

The *affinity to hydrophilic and hydrophobic surfaces* is particularly useful in the hydrophilization of a wide range of substances, ranging from hydrophobic tablet cores – to permit sugar or film-coating, to medical plastics.

The ability to form *complexes* with such a large number of substances is a special feature of polyvinylpyrrolidone (Section 2.2.7). The complexes formed are almost always soluble and are stable only in an acid medium. This property can be used to increase the solubility of drugs in liquid dosage forms, as in the case of povidone-iodine. In solid dosage forms, the ability to form complexes is used to increase bioavailability. A reduction in the local toxicity of certain drugs can also be achieved by complexation with povidone. A special use for the complexation properties lies in the stabilization of proteins and enzymes in diagnostics.

The *thickening properties* (Section 2.2.3) are used in oral and topical liquid dosage forms, e.g. syrups and suspensions.

Table 56. General properties of povidone in pharmaceuticals

- Solubility in all conventional solvents
- Adhesive and binding power
- Film formation
- Affinity to hydrophilic and hydrophobic surfaces
- Ability to form complexes
- Availability in different average molecular weights
- Thickening properties

Table 57. Main applications of povidone in the pharmaceuticals industry

Function	Pharmaceutical form
Binder	Tablets, capsules, granules
Bioavailability enhancer	Tablets, capsules, granules, pellets, suppositories, transdermal systems
Film former	Ophthalmic solutions, tablet cores, medical plastics
Solubilizer	Oral, parenteral and topical solutions
Taste masking	Oral solutions, chewing tablets
Lyophilisation agent	Injectables, oral lyophilisates
Suspension stabilizer	Suspensions, instant granules, dry syrups
Hydrophilizer	Medical plastics, sustained release forms, suspensions
Adhesive	Transdermal systems, adhesive gels
Stabilizer	Enzymes in diagnostics, different forms
Intermediate	Povidone-Iodine as active ingredient
Toxicity reduction	Injectables, oral preparations etc.

Povidone is available in grades of *different average molecular weight* (Section 2.2.6), as the above properties almost all depend on the molecular weight, to a greater or lesser extent:

With increasing molecular weight, the dissolution rate of povidone grades decreases, while the adhesive power, the viscosity and often also the ability to form complexes increase. The rate of elimination from the organism after parenteral administration decreases with increasing molecular weight.

This dependence of the properties on the molecular weight makes it possible to provide the optimum grade for each dosage form or formulation and to achieve the optimum effect.

2.4.2 Binders for tablets, granules and hard gelatin capsules

2.4.2.1 *General notes on tabletting and on povidone as a binder*

The main area of application of povidone K 25, 30 and 90 is as a binder for tablets and granules, as well as hard gelatin capsules. Its use is independent of whether wet or dry granulation or direct compression is used (Fig. 36), as povidone acts as a binder in all these processes.

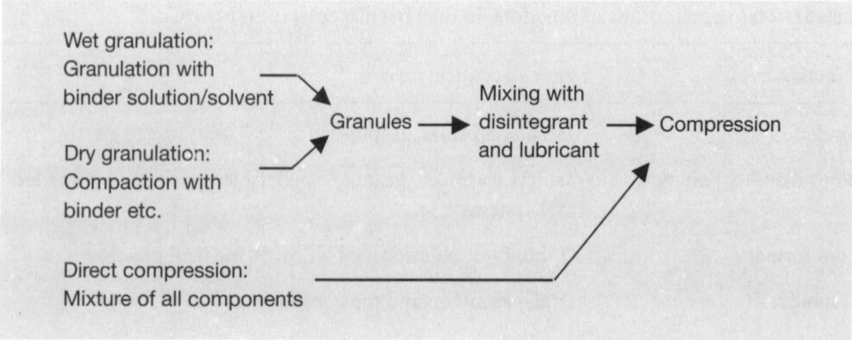

Fig. 36. General methods of tabletting

Table 58. Usual concentrations as a binder

Povidone type	Concentration in tablet/granules
Povidone K 25	2–5%
Povidone K 30	2–5%
Povidone K 90	1–3%

Table 59. The influence of different povidone types in a concentration of 5 % on the particle size distribution of a corn-starch granulate obtained by wet granulation

	Without	Povidone K 25	Povidone K 30	Povidone K 90
Fraction < 50 µm	> 99%	28%	27%	23%
50 µm – 100 µm	< 1%	23%	22%	10%
Fraction > 250 µm	–	44%	44%	61%

The usual concentrations in which povidone is used as a binder in tablets and granules are given in Table 58.

As povidone K 90 is a stronger binder than povidone K 25 or povidone K 30, the concentration given in Table 58 is about half that of the other two grades. This is confirmed in Table 59, which shows that the coarse fraction of a granulate increases and the fine fraction is reduced to a greater extent with povidone K 90 than with the other two types of lower mean molecular weight, for the same concentration.

It can also be seen from Table 59 that there is hardly any difference in the particle sizes of the granules produced with povidone K 25 and povidone K 30. A similar relationship is found when the hardness of placebo tablets is compared. It can be seen from Figs. 37 and 38 that there is no major difference between povidone K 25 and povidone K 30, even over a range of compression forces, while povidone K 90 gives significantly harder tablets.

Because of their good solubility in water, povidone hardly any adverse effect on the disintegration time of tablets in which they are used. Fig. 39 shows how the disintegration time of calcium hydrogen phosphate placebo tablets with 3% povi-

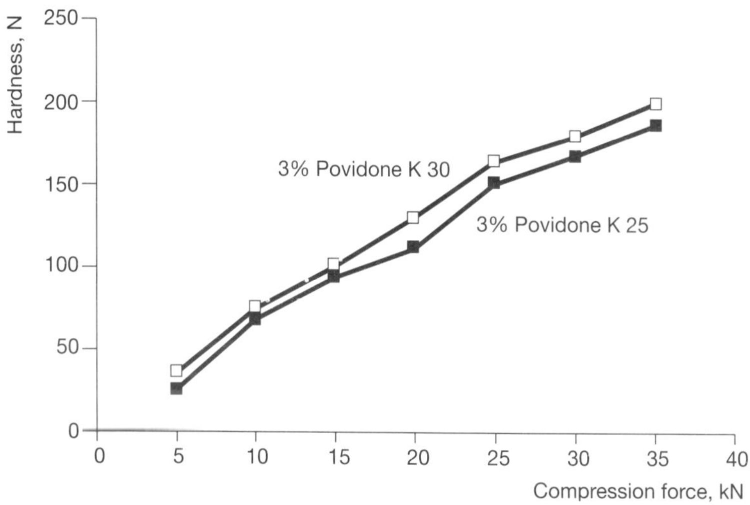

Fig. 37. Influence of compression force on the hardness of calcium hydrogen phosphate tablets (wet granulation)

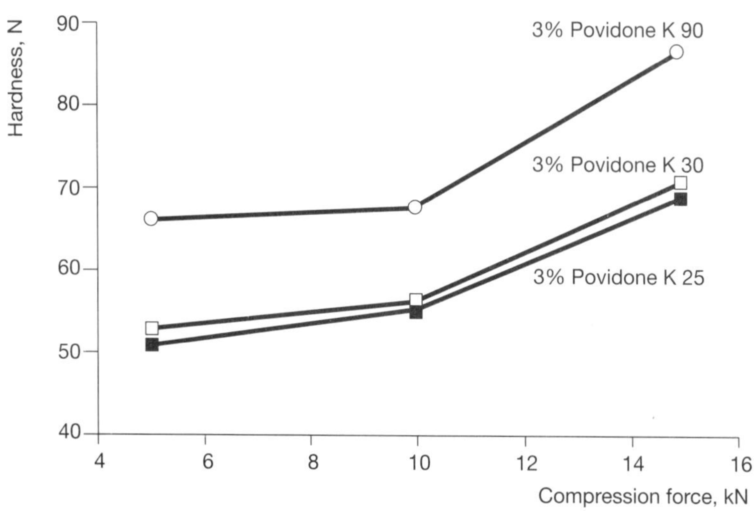

Fig. 38. Influence of compression force on the hardness of lactose monohydrate tablets (wet granulation)

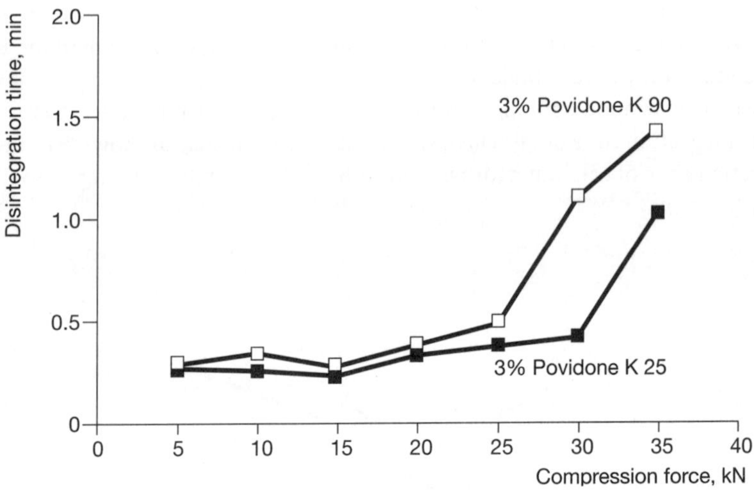

Fig. 39. Influence of the compression force on the disintegration time of calcium hydrogen phosphate placebo tablets with 3% crospovidone as disintegrant

done K 25 as binder remains more or less the same up to a high compression force of 30 kN. With 3% povidone K, it remains equally fast up to a compression force of 25 kN.

2.4.2.2
Production of tablets by wet granulation

Wet granulation is still the most widely used technique for preparing a tabletting mixture. There are at least four different variations of the procedure (Table 60).

Water is nowadays the most commonly used solvent. Sometimes, if water cannot be used, as with effervescent tablets, active ingredients that are prone to hydrolysis etc., ethanol or 2-propanol are used as solvents, though fluidized bed granulation technology is preferred.

Table 60. Methods of wet granulation with a binder

1. Granulation of the active substance (+ filler) with a binder solution.
2. Granulation of the active substance (+ filler)-binder mixture with the pure solvent.
3. Granulation of a mixture of the active substance (+ filler) and a portion of the binder with a solution of the remaining binder.
4. Granulation of the active substance (+ filler) with the solution of a portion of the binder followed by dry addition of the remaining binder to the finished granules.

There are a number of factors that dictate which of the methods in Table 60 must be used. With many formulations, Method 1 gives tablets with a shorter disintegration time and quicker release of the active substance than Method 2 [314]. In many cases, Method 1 gives somewhat harder tablets than Method 2. Method 3 in Table 60 is useful if Method 1 cannot be used, as when the tabletting mixture lacks the capacity for the quantity of liquid required (Table 66). If the disintegration time of a tablet presents a problem, it is worth trying Method 4, mixing in about a third of the binder together with lubricant and, last of all, the disintegrant.

Methods 2 and 3 have proved best for drugs of high solubility, as the quantity of liquid can be kept small to avoid clogging the granulating screens.

Wet granulation with povidone K 25, povidone K 30 or povidone K 90 generally gives harder granules with better flow properties than with other binders [64–77, 107, 234, 241, 243, 275, 503] with lower friability and higher binding strength. Fig. 40 shows a comparison with cellulose derivatives in placebo tablets, and it can be seen in Fig. 41 that povidone K 30 gives more than the double hardness of hydrochlorothiazide tablets in comparison to maltodextrin [527]. However, not only the hardness or friability can be better, povidone also promotes the dissolution of the active ingredient. As can be seen in Fig. 42, acetaminophen (paracetamol) tablets with 4% povidone K 90 as binder release the drug more quickly than tablets with gelatin or hydroxypropylcellulose as binder, even though the povidone tablets are harder. Similar results were obtained with 0.6 or 1.0% of povidone K 90 or hydroxypropylcellulose [544].

Povidone can be used in all the current wet granulation techniques, including fluidized bed granulation [82, 156, 425] and extrusion-spheronisation [157,

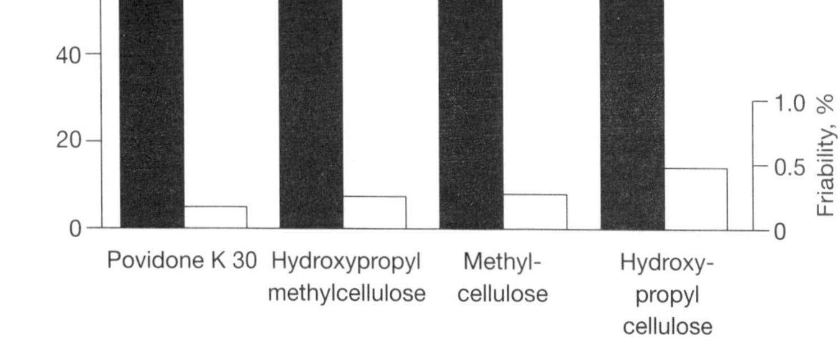

Fig 40. Hardness and friability of calcium phosphate placebo tablets with 3% binder (wet granulation)

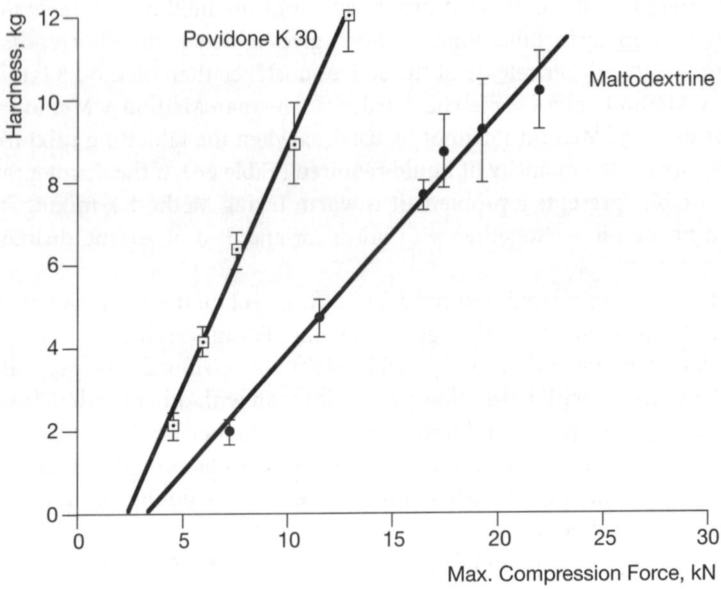

Fig. 41. Influence of 5% maltodextrine (Lycatab® DSH) and povidone on the hardness of hydrochlorothiazide tablets [527].

Lycatab® is a registered tradename of Roquettes Frères SA, Lestrem, France

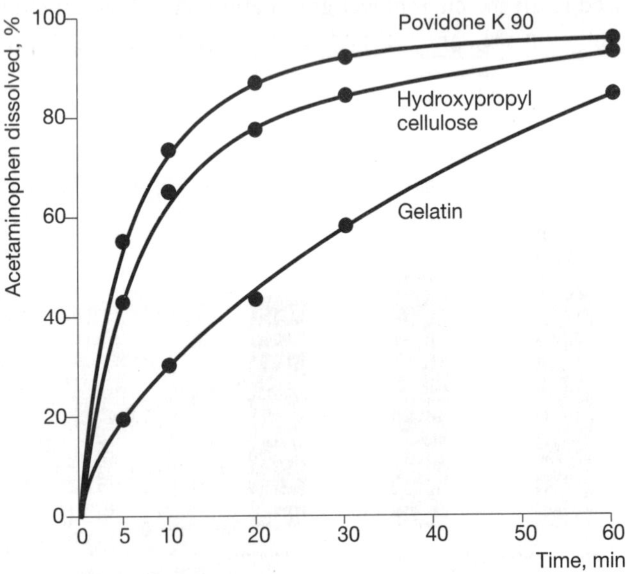

Fig. 42. Dissolution characteristics of acetaminophen tablets containing 4% binder [425]

591, 602] or drying by microwave radiation [561], though with povidone K 90, the viscosity of the granulating solution can be critical if the technique used does not permit the use of an adequate quantity of solvent. In difficult cases, it is actually possible to improve the properties of the granulate by using granulating solutions containing a mixture of different povidone grades instead of a single grade [218] or a mixture with HPMC [581]. The addition of low-molecular polyethylene glycol to the granulating solution can improve the plasticity of the granulate [78–81].

As already shown in Table 59, particle size is increased by granulation with povidone. This increase also depends on the quantity of povidone. If microcrystalline cellulose is granulated in a range of concentrations of 0–4% of the binder by Methods 1 and 2 in Table 60, the increase in particle size of the cellulose granulate is much the same in both methods (Fig. 43).

However, it has been possible to demonstrate in the production of caffeine tablets, that povidone K 25 increases the particle size and bulk density of the granulate, giving it better flow properties and reducing the friability of the tablets [400].

In wet granulation, the quantity of solvent, usually water, has a definite influence on the tablet properties. Increasing the amount of water as granulation liquid gave naproxen tablets with a significantly higher dissolution rate [534], ace-

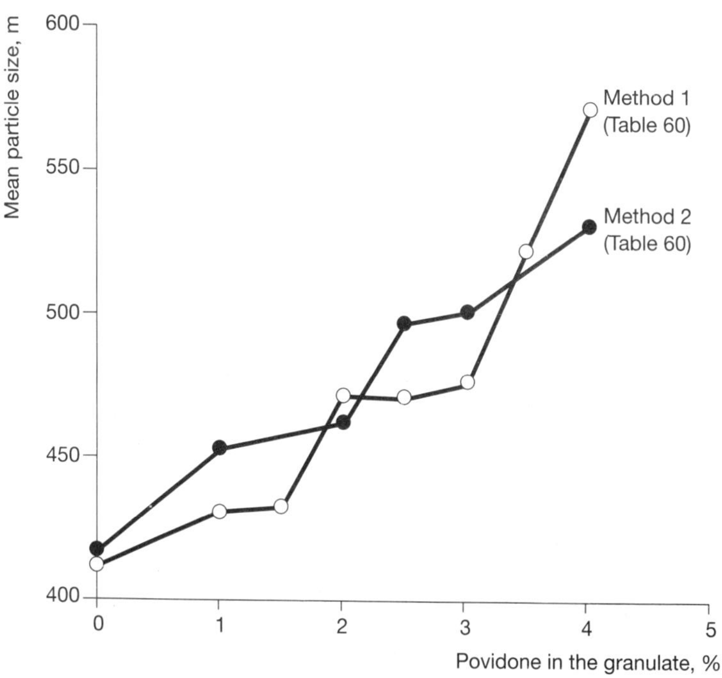

Fig. 43. Increase in the mean particle size of a cellulose granulate as a function of the binder concentration [362]

taminophen granules that were coarser and had better flowability [549], and calcium hydrogen phosphate tablets with shorter disintegration times (Table 47). The hardness of the calcium tablets remained unchanged if the particle size of the binder was the same. The amount of granulation liquid showed a stronger effect on to the particle size and drug release than the percentage of povidone in phenylbutazone pellets manufactured by extrusion-spheronisation [157] and had an influence on the yield [591].

The optimum quantity of solvent can best be determined from the power consumption of the granulator, though it must be noted that this can vary considerably, even with the same active substance, depending on its origin [484] (Table 61). For the comparison with copovidone see Section 4.4.2.2.

Table 61. Influence of the quantity of granulation liquid (water) on the tablet properties

Povidone K 90	Hardness		Disintegration time	
(% per tablet)	31 ml H_2O*	52 ml H_2O*	31 ml H_2O*	52 ml H_2O*
1.5%	94 N	99 N	105 min	34 min
3.0%	114 N	110 N	118 min	28 min

* In each case, the quantity of water relates to 515 g of $CaHPO_4$ granules

Table 62. Rifampicin tablets (450 mg) [615]

I	Rifampicin	450 g
	Corn starch	58 g
II	Povidone K 90	9 g
	Isopropanol	50 ml
III	Crospovidone	15 g
	Stearic acid	10 g
	Magnesium stearate	2 g
	Aerosil® 200	2 g

Granulate Mixture I with Solution II, dry, sieve and mix in the components of III, then press into tablets on a rotary tablet press using a low compression force.

Properties of tablets obtained in the laboratory:

Weight:	550 mg
Diameter:	12 mm
Hardness:	95 N
Disintegration time (gastric juice):	1–2 min
Friability:	0.6 %
Dissolution in 0.1 N hydrochloric acid according to USP:	15 min: 86%
	30 min: 90%

Aerosil® is a registered trademark of Degussa AG, Düsseldorf, Germany

The function and use of povidone K 30 and povidone K 90 as binders for wet granulation is shown in Tabs. 62–64 for several tablet formulations with drugs, developed on a laboratory scale. They were prepared by Method 1 in Table 60.

Povidone K 25 and povidone K 30 are very good binders for effervescent tablets, as they dissolve rapidly in water to form a clear solution. This particularly applies to effervescent vitamin tablets, e.g. ascorbic acid tablets [368 b]. Tables 65 and 66 give formulations for ranitidine effervescent tablets and multivitamin effervescent tablets as typical examples that were developed on a laboratory scale. For the granulation of multivitamin preparations, it is always preferable to use a fluidized bed.

In Table 66, the vitamin A palmitate should be replaced by a more modern water-dispersible vitamin A acetate dry powder, for better stability.

An interesting application for povidone as a binder lies in the wet granulation of auxiliaries in the manufacture of direct compression auxiliaries (e.g. [376], Table 67) and in the granulation of active substances for direct compression.

Active substances that are marketed in the pre-granulated form for direct compression are almost always substances that are difficult to press into tablets and/or are prone to hydrolysis. Typical examples are the vitamins and acetaminophen [540]. Table 68 contains details on the production of ascorbic acid for direct compression, which is granulated with povidone K 30 as binder in a fluidized bed granulator.

Table 63. Pyrazinamide tablets (500 mg) [615]

I	Pyrazinamide	500 g
	Corn starch	50 g
II	Povidone K 30	20 g
	Water	approx. 200 ml
III	Crospovidone	10–11 g
	Magnesium stearate	6 g

Granulate Mixture I with Solution II, sieve, dry and mix in the components of III, then press into tablets on a rotary tablet press with a low compression force.

Properties of tablets obtained in the laboratory:

Weight:	610 mg
Diameter:	12 mm
Hardness:	131 N
Disintegration time (gastric juice):	3 min
Friability:	0.25 %
Dissolution in water (USP method):	15 min: 78%
	30 min: 96%

Table 64. Alpha-methyldopa tablet cores (275 mg) [615]

I	Alpha-methyldopa	275 g
	Lactose monohydrate	55 g
II	Povidone K 30	15 g
	Isopropanol (or water)	80 ml
III	Crospovidone	8 g
	Magnesium stearate	2 g

Granulate Mixture I with Solution II, dry, sieve and mix in the components of III, then press into tablets on a rotary press with a medium compression force (approx. 15 kN).

Properties of tablets obtained in the laboratory:

Weight:	361 mg
Hardness:	118 N
Disintegration time (gastric juice):	5 min
Friability:	0 %
Dissolution in 0.1 N hydrochloric acid (USP method):	15 min: 77% 30 min: 98%

Table 65. Ranitidine effervescent tablets [360]

I	Ranitidine hydrochloride	168 g
	Anhydrous monosodium citrate	840 g
	Sodium bicarbonate	836 g
	Saccharin sodium	11 g
II	Povidone K 30	40 g
	Ethanol 96%	q.s.
III	Lemon flavour (powder)	25 g
	Sodium benzoate, siliconized (10%)	80 g

Granulate Mixture I with Solution II, dry, sieve and mix in III, then press into 2-g tablets.

It is essential to carry out the wet granulation of active substances that are prone to hydrolysis on a fluidized bed granulator, to preserve their stability. If an ascorbic acid granulate with 2.5% povidone and 2.5% crospovidone is produced as described in Table 68, and compared with a granulate of the same composition produced by traditional means (Diosna Mixer), only the granulate produced on the fluidized bed granulator proves stable. Figure 44 shows the change in colour of these two granulates after 6 months' storage at room temperature.

The results shown in Fig. 44 demonstrate clearly that reports of incompatibility of povidone with ascorbic acid in a number of publications are based on misinterpretations or the use of inappropriate methods.

Table 66. Multivitamin effervescent tablets [615]

1. Formulation

I	Thiamine mononitrate	13	g
	Riboflavin	4	g
	Pyridoxine hydrochloride	11	g
	Nicotinamide	66	g
	Calcium pantothenate	17	g
	Tartaric acid	360	g
	Sodium bicarbonate	550	g
	Sucrose, crystalline	300	g
	Sucrose, powder	300	g
	Povidone K 30	35	g
II	Povidone K 30	5	g
	2-Propanol	approx. 80	g
III	Riboflavin	6	g
	Ascorbic acid, powder	550	g
	Cyanocobalamin 0.1% gelatin dry powder	20	g
	Vitamin A palmitate 250 000 I.U./g dry powder CWD	12	g
	Vitamin E acetate dry powder SDG 50	60	g
	PEG 6000, powder	80	g
	Crospovidone	100	g

Granulate Mixture I with Solution II, in a fluidized bed granulator, if possible; dry, then mix with the components of III and press into tablets on a rotary tablet press with a relatively high compression force.

2. Properties of the tablets obtained in the laboratory

Weight:	2500	mg
Diameter:	20	mm
Hardness:	140	N
Disintegration time (gastric juice):	1–2	min
Friability:	1	%

3. Stability (vitamin loss after 12 months at 23 °C, HPLC methods)

Ascorbic acid:	8	%
Cyanocobalamin:	8	%
Vitamin A:	29	%
All other vitamins:	Not more than 6	%

Table 67. Composition of the Ludipress® direct compression auxiliary

Lactose monohydrate	93.0%
Povidone K 30	3.5%
Crospovidone	3.5%

Ludipress® is a registered trademark of BASF AG, Ludwigshafen, Germany

Table 68. Ascorbic acid granules for direct compression [369]

I	Ascorbic acid powder	1920 g
II	Povidone K 30	80 g
	Water	600 ml

Granulate the ascorbic acid (I) with an aqueous solution of povidone K 30 (II) in a 15-kg fluidized bed granulator under the following conditions:

Inlet air temperature:	60°C
Inlet air rate:	Maximum setting
Spray pressure:	2–3 bar
Spraying time:	8–10 min
Drying time:	5 min
Final water content:	< 0.5%

Stability:

After storage for 3 months at 40°C in airtight containers, the white colour of the product had not changed.

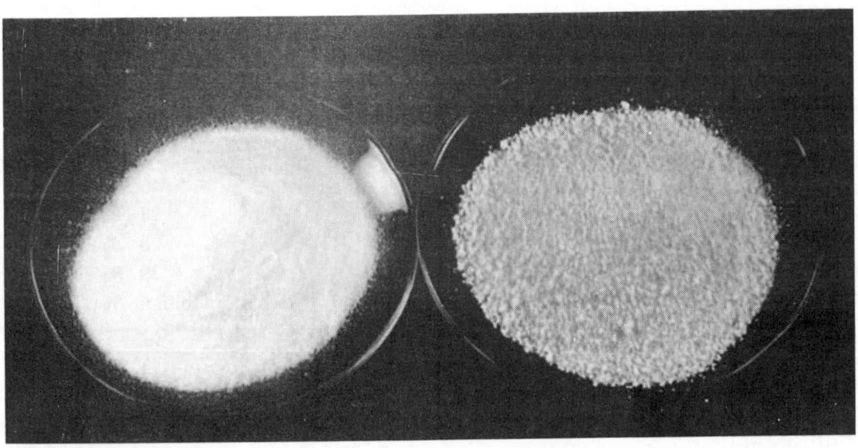

Fig. 44. The influence of different methods of wet granulation on the colour stability of an ascorbic acid granulate with povidone K 30 (after 6 months at room temperature)
Left: Fluidized bed granulate. *Right:* Diosna Mixer granulate

2.4.2.3
Production of tabletting mixtures by dry granulation

Dry granulation is less frequently used than wet granulation or direct compression in the preparation of tablets. The most widely known dry granulation technology is the roller compaction technique. A new tech-nology is the ultrasonic compaction [607]. It offers advantages when wet granulation would affect the stability, and when the physical properties of the drug do not allow direct compression.

Povidone is a very good binder for this type of granulation, too [324]. Ascorbic acid provides a typical example (Table 69).

The compacted powder described in Table 69 was pressed into tablets (see Table 70 for the formulation) and provided a preparation that hardly changed its colour during storage at room temperature over a period of 3 years.

Table 69. Roller compacted ascorbic acid-povidone mixture [367]

Ascorbic acid powder	96 %
Povidone K 30	3 %
Crospovidone (micronized)	1 %

Compact a homogeneous mixture of the three components and break up by forcing through a screen. Sieve off the coarse fraction.

Table 70. Ascorbic acid tablets from compacted powder with povidone K 30 [367]

Ascorbic acid compacted powder 96% (Table 69)	300.0 g
Microcrystalline cellulose	200.0 g
Polyethylene glycol 6000, powder	20.0 g
Talc	4.0 g
Aerosil® 200	0.5 g
Calcium arachinate	0.5 g

Mix all the components and press into tablets on a rotary tablet press with a relatively low compression force.

Properties of the tablets obtained in the laboratory:

Weight:	525 mg
Diameter:	12 mm
Hardness:	115 N
Disintegration (gastric juice):	90 s
Friability:	< 0.1 %
Colour stability (23 °C):	Hardly any change over 3 years

2.4.2.4
Direct compression

Although most active substances are not in themselves suitable for direct compression in the concentrations required, this technique has recently grown in importance.

Not only substances with good compressibility can be used in direct compression (Table 71). Drug preparations – usually granules with a binder – that can be tabletted directly, as well as direct compression auxiliaries are available on the market for problem substances.

Povidone K 25 and povidone K 30 can be used for all three types of direct compression of Table 71 but the more plastic and less hygroscopic copovidone would be better for this technique. Many direct compression auxiliaries, or grades of active substances suitable for direct compression already contain a binder such as povidone. In such cases, little or no further povidone need be added.

Table 71. Different forms of direct compression

Properties of the drug	Type of direct compression
Directly compressible in adequate concentrations	The active substance is tabletted with the usual auxiliaries
Not directly compressible in the desired concentration with the usual auxiliaries	A direct compression agent, is used
	Direct compression granules of the active substance are used.

Table 72. Direct compression of metronidazole tablets [615] (compression force: 25 kN)

Metronidazole	200 g
Microcrystalline cellulose	200 g
Povidone K 30	6 g
Crospovidone	10 g
Aerosil® 200	5 g
Magnesium stearate	5 g
Properties of the tablets obtained in the laboratory:	
Weight	426 mg
Diameter	12 mm
Hardness	133 N
Disintegration time (gastric juice)	1–2 min
Friability	<0.1 %

Table 73. Direct compression of vitamin B complex tablets

Thiamine mononitrate	25 g
Riboflavin	25 g
Nicotinamide	50 g
Calcium-D-pantothenate	40 g
Pyridoxine hydrochloride	16 g
Cyanocobalamin 0.1% in gelatin	16 g
Microcrystalline cellulose	175 g
Kovidone K 30	16 g
Aerosil® 200	6 g

Properties of the tablets obtained in the laboratory:

Weight	365 mg
Diameter	12 mm
Hardness	171 N
Disintegration (gastric juice)	10 min
Friability	0 %

Stability of Vitamin B_1: 17% loss in activity after 6 months at 40 °C [368a]

In direct compression, the moisture content of the tabletting mixture is important, though under normal conditions, the usual residual quantity of water in povidone already provides an adequate binding effect between the particles.

To demonstrate the application of povidone in the direct compression technique, metronidazole tablets (Table 72) and vitamin B complex tablets (Table 73) were tested in the laboratory.

2.4.2.5
Granules, hard gelatin capsules

The granulation and binding properties of povidone used in tabletting obviously also make these products suitable for the production of granules as a dosage form. There are various types of granules (Table 74), for which the various granulation techniques given in Table 60 can be used.

The drugs most frequently incorporated in *instant granules* are antacids and vitamins. Table 75 gives details of a magaldrate instant granule formulation developed in the laboratory, as an example of this dosage form.

Vitamins are very often incorporated in *effervescent granules*. Table 76 gives details of a multivitamin effervescent granule formulation developed in the laboratory. The chemical stability of this guide formulation has not yet been tested.

The most important reasons for using granules to fill *hard gelatin capsules* are to improve the flow properties and to reduce dust formation in the filling machine. If the filling is free-flowing, it can be metered with greater conformity into the individual capsules.

Table 74. Different types of granules

- Instant granules
- Effervescent granules
- Chewable granules
- Dry syrup granules
- Granules for filling hard gelatin capsules

Table 75. Magaldrate instant granules [615]

I	Magaldrate	10.0 g
	Micronized crospovidone (low bulk density)	8.0 g
	Sorbitol, crystalline	5.0 g
	Orange flavouring	1.0 g
II	Povidone K 90	1.0 g
	Coconut flavouring	0.1 g
	Banana flavouring	0.1 g
	Saccharin sodium	0.02 g
	Water	approx. 7 ml

Granulate Mixture I with Solution II, sieve and dry.

To a certain extent, these arguments also apply to granules in other dosage forms, particularly when they are packaged as individual portions in sachets.

Further examples of formulations for instant granules are described in Chapter 3, under Section 3.4.4.3.

Table 76. Multivitamin effervescent granules (3–4 g = 1 RDA) [615]

I	Thiamine mononitrate	2.6 g
	Riboflavin	3.0 g
	Nicotinamide	11.0 g
	Pyridoxine hydrochloride	2.5 g
	Calcium-D-pantothenate	15.0 g
	Ascorbic acid	200.0 g
	Citric acid	500.0 g
	Sucrose	1300.0 g
	Fructose	800.0 g
	Micronized crospovidone (low bulk density)	200.0 g
	Cyclamate sodium	20.0 g
	Saccharin sodium	1.0 g
	Flavouring	250.0 g
II	Povidone K 30	150.0 g
	Isopropanol or ethanol	350.0 g
III	Vitamin A acetate dry powder 325 000 CWD	15.0 g
	Vitamin D3 dry powder 100 000 CWD	8.0 g
	Vitamin E acetate dry powder SD 50	21.0 g
	Cyanocobalamin 0.1% in gelatin	6.6 g
	Sodium bicarbonate	400.0 g

Granulate Mixture I with Solution II in a fluidized bed granulator, dry, sieve and mix with III. Thoroughly dry before packaging.

2.4.3 Improvement of the dissolution rate and bioavailability of drugs

2.4.3.1 *Physical mixtures with povidone*

One problem with many of the active substances used today is their poor solubility in water and their limited bioavailability. One of the simplest means of improving the bioavailability of an active substance is to improve its dissolution by adding solubilizing agents, such as povidone. It forms water-soluble complexes with many active substances (see Sections 2.2.7 and 2.4.5). With some such substances, it may be sufficient to produce a physical mixture. Fig. 45 shows the improvement in the dissolution rate of reserpine achieved by simply mixing it with an excess of povidone K 30. For the mixture with indomethacin see Section 3.4.3.1. Similar results can be expected with the drugs listed in Section 2.4.5. That this effect also applies to finished preparations can be seen for phenytoin tablets in Fig. 52 [326]. The bioavailability of peroral gidazepam is increased by the addition of povidone too [536].

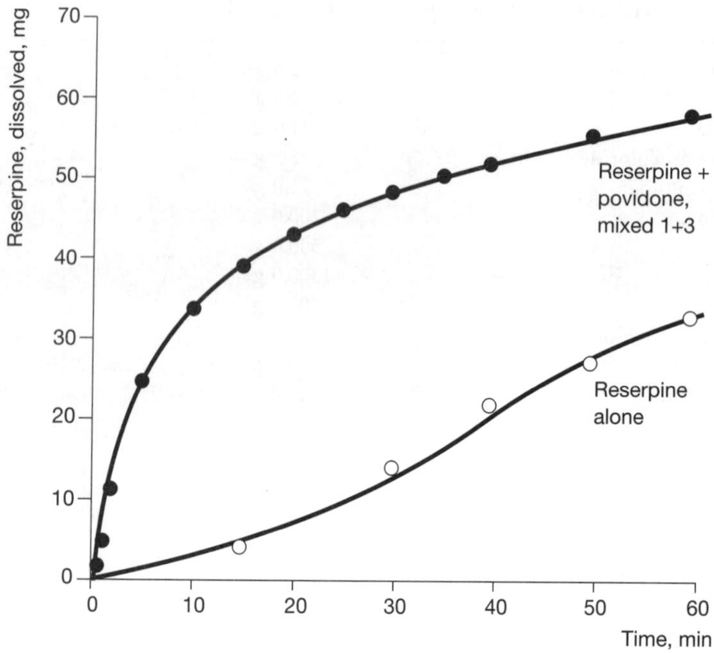

Fig. 45. Dissolution of reserpine [27]

2.4.3.2
Solid solutions/solid dispersions

If it is not possible to improve the bioavailability of a substance as desired by the addition of a solubilizing agent, this is frequently because the surface area of the crystals of active ingredient exposed to the solvent is too small. It is therefore necessary to increase the surface area, to accelerate dissolution. The first "solid dispersions" with antibiotics in povidone were described in the literature in about 1960 [49, 60]. In solid solutions and dispersions the active substance is embedded in a hydrophilic carrier to improve its bioavailability. The difference between a solid solution and a solid dispersion can be defined in terms of the state of the active substance. In a solid solution, it is present in an amorphous molecular form, while in a solid dispersion it is in the form of crystals that must be as fine as possible.

Povidone is an excellent auxiliary for the manufacture of effective solid solutions and dispersions as it

- possesses excellent hydrophilization properties,
- is available in different molecular weights for different viscosities,
- forms water-soluble complexes with many drugs, in contrast to most other carrier materials, and
- is almost universally soluble.

Table 77. Nomenclature and techniques of manufacture for solid solutions and dispersions

Technique	Designation of the solid solution/solid dispersion
Solvent method:	
- Spray-drying	Spray-embedded preparation
- Normal drying, Vacuum-drying	Coprecipitate, coevaporate
- Freeze-drying, Lyophilization	Lyophilisate
- Spray-drying of suspension	Spray-dried suspension [538]
Cogrinding, roll-mixing	Trituration
Extrusion, melt extrusion	Extrudate

This is why more than 150 drugs in solid solutions and dispersions with povidone have been described in the literature between 1960 and 2002.

Manufacture of solid solutions:
Various techniques can be used to produce solid solutions and dispersions. The nomenclature for these is varied and not uniform, as can be seen from Table 77.

Unlike other polymers such as polyethylene glycol, melted povidone is almost not used as an embedding matrix for drugs, except in melt extrusion, because of its high melting point (over 180 °C with decomposition).

Coprecipitates:
The most frequently used method of manufacturing solid solutions and dispersions with povidone has up to now been the solvent method. In this, the active substance and povidone are dissolved together in a solvent and this is subsequently evaporated in an oven, under vacuum or sometimes by spray-drying.

If possible, ethanol is used as the solvent. Unfortunately, its solvent power is inadequate for a number of active substances. However, as the active substance must be completely dissolved to distribute the drug in the carrier in a very fine crystalline to amorphous form, it is then necessary to resort to the use of another organic solvent such as chloroform.

Triturations:
As it is nowadays often no longer practical to use organic solvents, it is recommended to select a different technique such as roll-mixing or comilling with povidone. That this method is also capable of producing an amorphous distribution of phenytoin and many other active substances is shown in Fig. 46 and in Table 78. In which two roll-mixed preparations are com-pared with the crystalline active substance and a solvent-coprecipitate by X-ray diffraction.

Table 78 shows that this milling or intimate mixing technique improves the dissolution and the bioavailability [353, 378, 438] of many active substances. All the

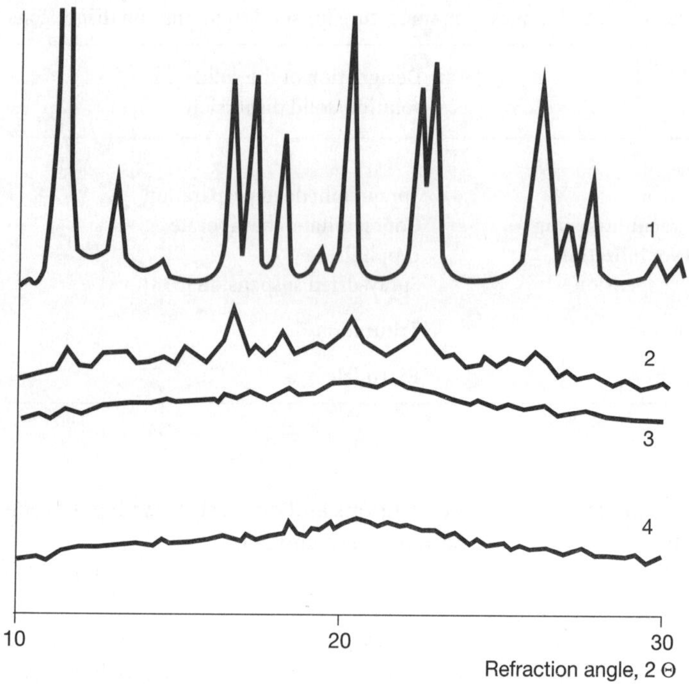

Fig. 46: Effect of the roll-mixing process on the crystallinity of phenytoin [226]:
1: Phenytoin without povidone
2: Phenytoin + povidone K 30 1 + 1
3: Phenytoin + povidone K 30 1 + 3
4: Phenytoin + povidone K 30 coprecipitate 1 + 3 (for comparison)

active substances were found to have an amorphous or at least partly amorphous structure in the mixtures, which indicates that they form complexes with povidone even in the absence of a solvent.

The physical stability of the mixtures tested [326, 352, 381, 432, 569] was found to be good, and no decrease in the dissolution rate was found after storage.

Povidone K 25 and povidone K 30 are suitable for comilling, while the average molecular weight of povidone K 90 could decrease under prolonged mechanical stress. As a rule, the mixtures are milled for one hour, though the best time must be determined individually for each active substance.

Ratio of active substance to povidone:
As can already be seen from Fig. 46, the ratio of the quantities of active substance and povidone is a further factor that influences the way in which the active substance is distributed in the matrix and therefore also the dissolution and bioavailability of the active substance. Although a 1 + 1 ratio already achieves a certain effect, it is only when the auxiliary is used in larger proportions, typically 1 + 3 to

Table 78. The effect of comilling or physically mixing active substances with povidone on their crystallinity and dissolution rate

Active substance	Crystallinity	Improvement in dissolution	Literature reference
Acridine	Amorphous	+	[429]
Amobarbital	Amorphous	+	[430]
Atenolol	Partly amorphous	+	[613]
Chlordiazepoxide	Partly amorphous	+	[254]
Chlormadinone acetate	n.d.	+	[378]
Clonazepam	Partly amorphous	+	[254]
Diacetylmidecamycin	Amorphous	n.d.	[432]
Diazepam	Partly amorphous	+	[254, 433]
Furosemide	Partly amorphous	+	[636]
Glibenclamide	(Partly) Amorphous	+	[572]
Griseofulvin	Amorphous	+	[351, 428, 436]
Hydrochlorothiazide	Partly amorphous	+	[550]
Ibuprofen	Amorphous	–	[557]
Indobufen derivative	Amorphous	+	[438]
Indomethacin	Amorphous	+	[351]
Kitasamycin	n.d.	+	[435]
Medazepam	Partly amorphous	+	[254]
Menadione	Amorphous	+	[429]
Mydecamycin	Amorphous	n.d.	[381]
Nifedipine	Amorphous	+	[251, 352]
Nitrazepam	Partly amorphous	+	[254]
Oestradiol	Amorphous	+	[592]
Oxytetracycline	Partly amorphous	+	[431]
Phenacetin	Amorphous	+	[350, 351, 434]
Phenothiazine	Amorphous	+	[429]
Phenytoin	Amorphous	+	[226]
Praziquantel	Amorphous	+	[610, 638]
Prednisolone	n.d.	+	[437]
Probucol	n.d.	+	[353]
Sulfathiazole	Amorphous	+	[551]
Theophylline	Partly amorphous	+	[569]

n.d. = not determined

1 + 10, that a molecular dispersion of the active substance in the carrier is obtained. Fig. 47 shows as an example the dissolution rate of sulfathiazole triturations with different quantities of povidone. Similar results were obtained with furosemide coprecipitates [259] and sulindac coprecipitates [604].

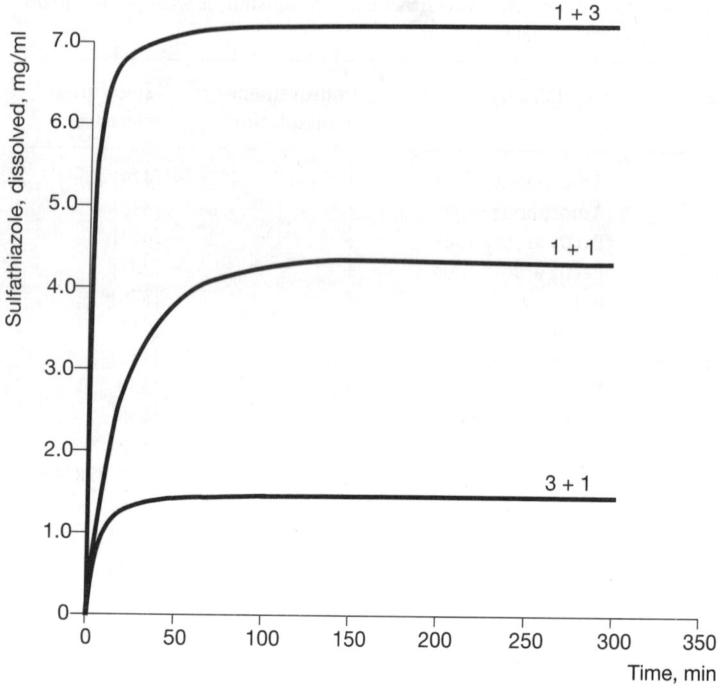

Fig. 47. Influence of the drug: povidone ratio on the dissolution of sulfathiazole triturations [551]

2.4.3.3
Influence of the molecular weight of the povidone type

The influence of the molecular weight of the povidone type on the dissolution and bioavailability of the embedded substance varies. It can generally be said only that the high-molecular povidone K 90 is less suitable, as it has a high viscosity in water and therefore dissolves too slowly, delaying dissolution of the active substance. Frequently, no major differences could be observed between the lower molecular weight grades, though with certain active substances, the dissolution rate was found to depend directly on the molecular weight of the povidone grade used [e.g. 44 b, 52 a, 306]. Naproxene [542] and sulfathiazole are such substances. Fig. 48 shows the dissolution of tablets made with 1 + 2 sulfathiazole coprecipitates with povidone of different molecular weights.

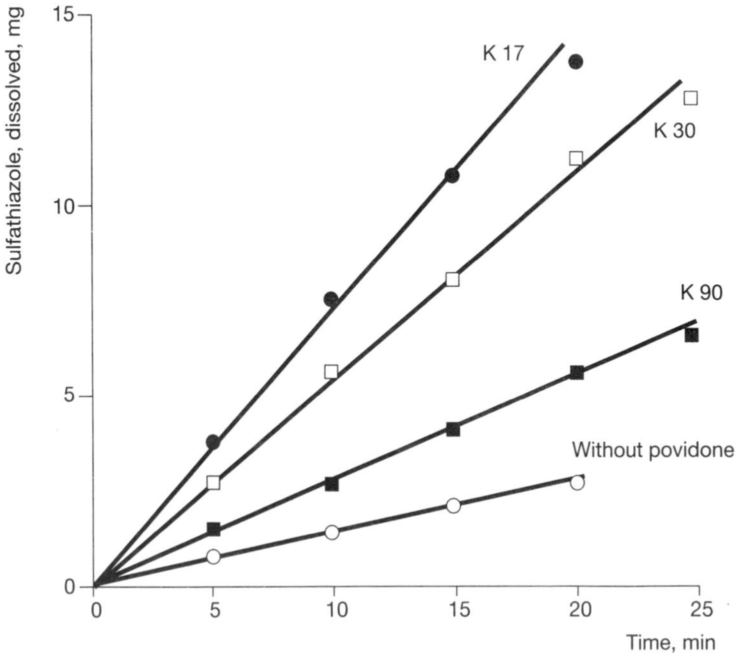

Fig. 48. Effect of the K-value of the povidone grade on the dissolution of tablets made with sulfathiazole coprecipitates [30a]

2.4.3.4
Bioavailability (in vivo)

Unfortunately, only relatively few of the many papers published on povidone deal with its influence on bioavailability in vivo. However, where results are available, they almost always show an improvement in bioavailability. Figs. 49 to 51 show the effect of coprecipitation with povidone on the bioavailability of different active substances administered by different routes. Fig. 49 shows, as a typical example, the oral bioavailability of a nifedipine coprecipitate in the rat, Fig. 50 shows the rectal bioavailability of a phenobarbital coprecipitate in rabbits, while Fig. 51 shows the effect of a hydrocortisone coprecipitate on the human skin after percutaneous administration. In all three cases, the same dose of the pure active substance without povidone was applied for reference.

With nifedipine, the plasma level of the coprecipitate reaches twice that of the pure substance after two hours and in the case of the phenobarbital suppositories, it even reaches three times the level of the pure active substance. Also in the case of Lonetil suppositories the use of a povidone coprecipitate could increase the resorption [146].

With hydrocortisone acetate, coprecipitation with povidone not only results in a doubling of the percutaneous effect after 30 minutes, the effect also lasts much

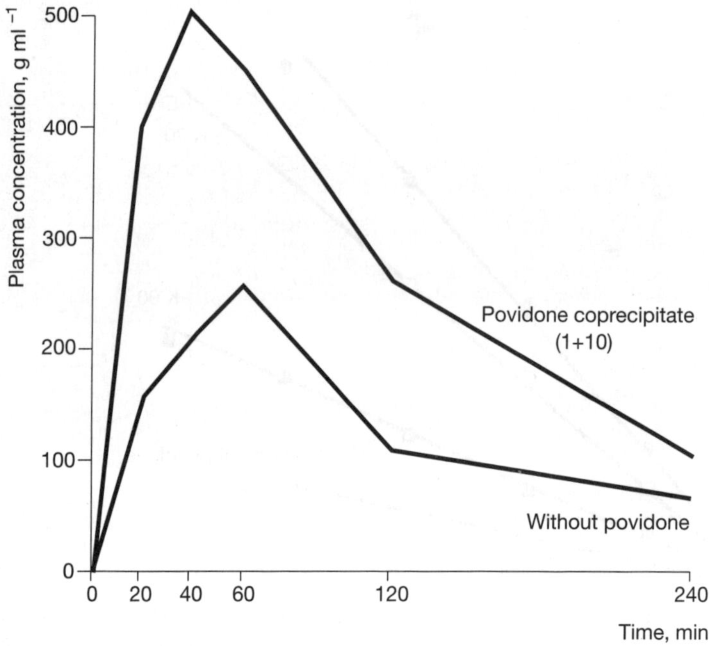

Fig. 49. Oral bioavailability of nifedipine in rats [253]

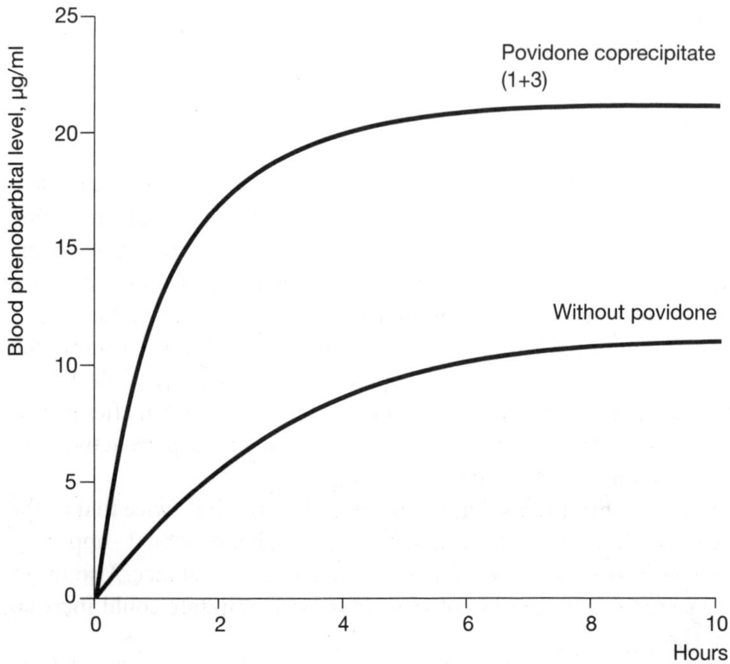

Fig. 50. Absorption of phenobarbital from suppositories in rabbits [224]

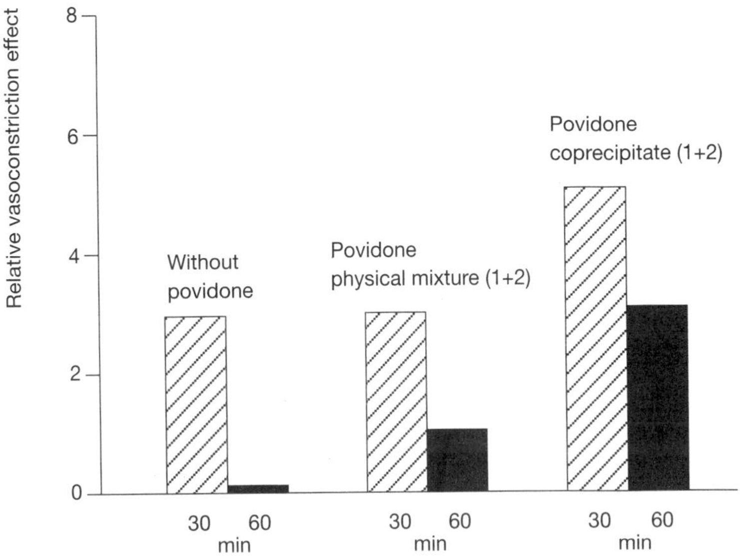

Fig. 51. Percutaneous effect of hydrocortisone acetate on the human skin [291]

longer. Without povidone, no further effect could be observed after 60 minutes, while with the coprecipitate, the effect was as strong after 1 hour as it was after 30 minutes for the pure active substance. Similar effects of povidone are observed with progesterone in rats [645] and in transdermal systems (see Section 2.4.8.2), in combination of hydrocortisone with beta-cyclodextrin [556] and combined with propylene glycol and oestradiol [567].

Also the ocular bioavailability of disulfiram could be strongly increased after the instillation of a 1% suspension of a solid dispersion with povidone K30 in the eye of rabbits [634].

The bioavailability of solid solutions and dispersions of active substances in povidone has mainly been tested in rabbits, dogs, rats and in man. Table 79 lists many of the active substances for which results are available in the literature.

2.4.3.5 Stability of solid solutions

As the active substance in a solid solution is in an amorphous state and therefore in a more energetic form, and as its surface area is much greater both in solid solutions and in solid dispersions, the question of its physical and chemical stability arises. The main criterion for physical stability is the extent of recrystallization, which can reduce the bioavailability of the active substance. Surprisingly, a survey of publications in which recrystallization and chemical stability have been investigated reveals only relatively few cases of instability. Table 80 contains a list of publications with stability data for solid solutions of drugs in povidone with a

Table 79. Publications on the improvement in bioavailability in vivo through the use of solid solutions and dispersions in povidone

Active substance	Man	Rabbit	Rat	Dog	Other
Acronycine					[41], [363]
Azapropazone		[283], [284]			
Betamethasone dipropionate	[291]				
Chloramphenicol				[45]	[230]
Chlormadinone acetate			[378]		
Chlorothiazide			[285]		
Chlorpropamide		[233], [234]			
Cyclosporine			[575]		
Dicumarol		[209]			
Digitoxin			[47b]		
Dihydroergotamine			[379]		
Dihydroergotoxine	[280]				
Drotaverine	[286]				
Floctafenine		[283], [284]			
Furosemide	[287]				
Gentamycin			[336]		
Glafenine		[283], [284]			
Glibenclamide			[288]		
Gliquidone	[279]				
Gossypol acetate					[289]
Griseofulvin				[290]	
Hexobarbital				[37]	
Hydrochlorothiazide	[53], [361]				
Hydrocortisone acetate	[291]				
Kanamycin			[336]		
Lonetil			[146]		
Lorazepam			[292]		
Mefenamic acid	[366]	[283], [284], [293]			
Nabilone	[294]			[294]	
Nifedipine		[295], [299], [358]	[253]	[205], [297]	[298]
Nitrofurantoin	[300]				
Nystatin					[301]
Oxolinic acid	[302], [303]				
Phenobarbital		[224]			
Phenytoin	[25], [150], [303]	[184], [304]			
Probucol		[353]			
Reserpine		[224]	[47a], [305]		
Rifampicin	[270]		[270]		
Sulfamethoxazole	[194]				
Sulfisoxazole	[145], [306]	[261]			
Tetracycline	[274]				
Tinidazole			[292]		
Tolbutamide		[111]	[63]		
Tyrothricin					[49]

Table 80. Publications on the stability results of solid solutions/dispersions of drugs in povidone compared with the pure drugs

Drug	Chemical stability Good	Chemical stability Inferior	Physical stability Good	Physical stability Inferior
Amoxicillin		[292], [355]		
Bromcip	[538]			
Chlordiazepoxide		[104]		
Chlorthalidone			[308]	
Clonazepam			[149a]	
Colecalciferol	[309]			
Diacetylmidecamycin			[432]	
Diazepam	[481]		[481]	
Dihydroergotamine methanesulfonate			[310]	
Drotaverine			[286]	
Ethylestrenol		[311]		
Flunitrazepam			[149a]	
Furosemide	[259], [265]		[178], [259], [265]	
Gliquidone			[614]	
Griseofulvin			[588]	[312]
Hydrocortisone	[313]		[295], [313]	
Hydroflumethiazide			[315], [316]	
Indomethazin		[513]		
Iomeglamic acid			[317]	
Ketoconazol			[643]	
Lonetil	[318]		[318]	
Lorazepam	[292]			
Lynestrenol		[311]		
Medazepam	[104]			
Mefruside			[319]	
Mydecamycin			[381]	
Nabilone			[294]	
Nifedipine	[135], [205], [297], [321]		[321], [352], [576]	[135], [205], [297], [322]
Nitrazepam			[149a], [323]	
Nitrofurantoin	[300]			
Oxodipine			[508]	
Phenobarbital			[314]	
Phenytoin	[326]		[31], [326]	
Prostaglandin	[327]			
Reserpine	[387]			
Salbutamol sulfate	[292], [328]		[328]	
Sulfamethizole			[61]	
Sulfisoxazole				[61]
Sulindac			[604]	
Testosterone			[52a]	
Tinidazole		[292]		

brief assessment of the results for both the chemical and the physical stability. A negative influence of the storage on the release was reported for ibuprofen.

One substance that has been subjected to a very long stability test, in a coprecipitate with povidone K 30 (1+9), is phenytoin. Its dissolution rate was practically the same after two years (Figs. 52 and 53).

2.4.3.6
Practical application in formulations

In spite of the many papers published on them and the often major improvements in bioavailability and the stability they provide, solid solutions and dispersions in povidone have up to now only found use in a few commercial products. Tables 81 and 82 show how phenytoin and nifedipine, for example, can be processed relatively straightforwardly in the form of a physical mixture or coprecipitate with povidone. Cyclosporine, oxodipine and spironolactone tablets or norethindrone suppositories are further examples [508, 533, 566, 575]. It is interesting to compare the dissolution data for phenytoin after manufacture and after two years' storage at room temperature in Figs. 52 and 53: no major difference can be seen.

The difference found between the two nifedipine tablet formulations in Table 82 stems from the way in which the coprecipitate is produced. In Formulation No. 1 it is produced separately and subsequently pressed together with a further granulate. In Formulation No. 2, the coprecipitate is formed on the surface of the cellu-

Table 81. Tablet formulation with phenytoin and povidone [326]

Formulation:

I	Phenytoin	10 mg
	Povidone K 30	90 mg
II	Corn starch	7 mg
	Lactose	3 mg

Production:
Method I (physical mixture):
Prepare Mixtures I and II, mix and press into tablets.

Method II (coprecipitate):
Dissolve phenytoin and povidone K 30 together in an organic solvent, evaporate this to dryness and mix the resulting coprecipitate with II, then press into tablets.

Properties of the tablets:

	Method I	Method II
Weight:	110 mg	110 mg
Diameter:	6 mm	6 mm
Disintegration time (after manufacture):	7 min	8 min
Disintegration time (after 2 years):	7–8 min	10 min

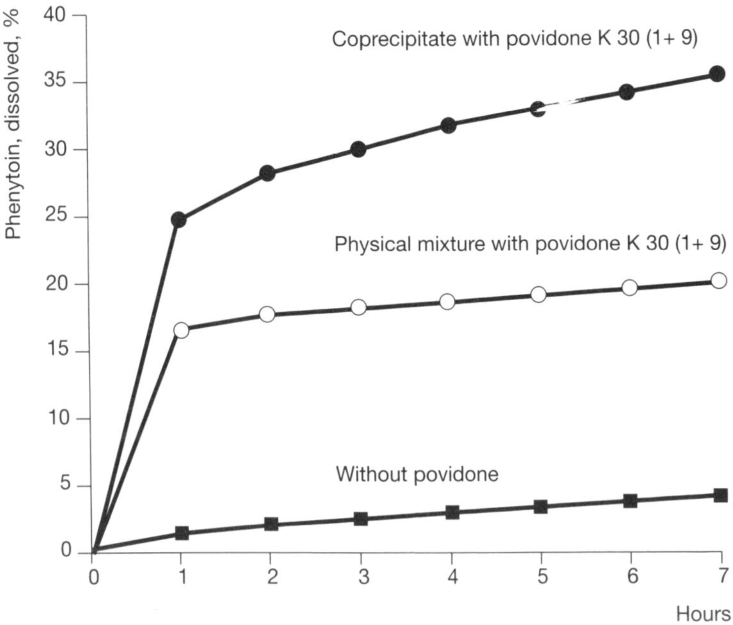

Fig. 52. Dissolution of phenytoin from tablets after manaufacture (formulation see Table 81) [326]

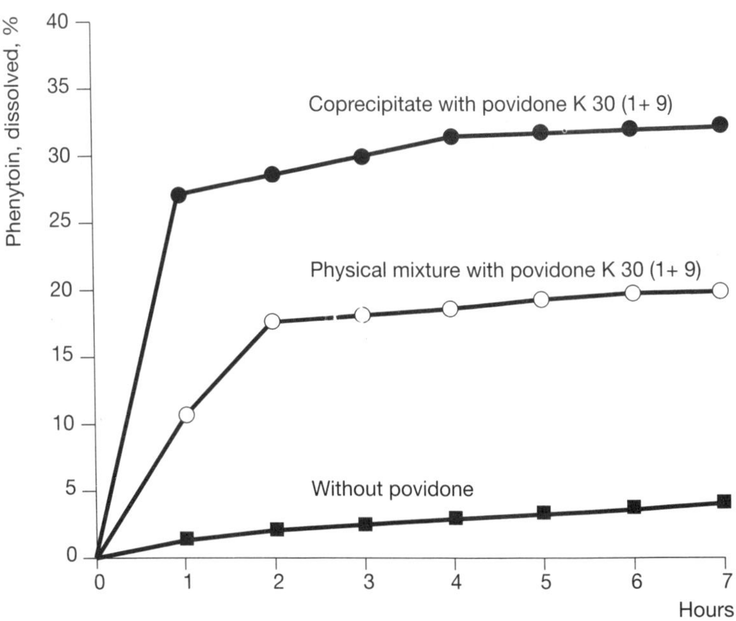

Fig. 53. Dissolution of phenytoin from tablets after storage for 2 years at 20 °C (formulation see Table 81)

Table 82. Nifedipine tablets made from coprecipitates with povidone [240 b]

	Formulation	No. 1	No. 2
I	Nifedipine	100 g	100 g
	Povidone K 25	400 g	400 g
II	Methylene chloride	1500 g	1800 g
III	Microcrystalline cellulose	1050 g	1050 g
	Corn starch	350 g	200 g
	Crospovidone	–	100 g
IV	Corn starch paste	50 g	–
V	Crospovidone	246 g	146 g
	Magnesium stearate	4 g	4 g

Manufacturing of Formulation No. 1:
Dissolve I in II, dry, sieve. Granulate III with IV, dry and sieve. Mix I/II, III/IV and V and press into tablets.

Manufacturing of Formulation No. 2:
Dissolve I in II and granulate with Mixture III. Dry, sieve, mix with V and press into tablets.

Properties of the tablets:

Formulation	No. 1	No. 2
Nifedipine content	10 mg (± 4.1%)	10 mg (±1.0%)
Weight	220 mg	220 mg
Dissolution rate (USP)	50% in 10 min	50% in 5 min

lose during granulation, an interesting variation. If all crospovidone was used intragranulary the dissolution was even faster.

There are two reasons why there are relatively few preparations based on coprecipitates. One is that it is necessary to use an organic solvent and the other is that an excess of the matrix is required to achieve the desired improvement in bioavailability.

With drugs that must be given in high doses, the large quantity of matrix limits the applications of solid solutions considerably, as it is difficult to produce tablets, capsules etc. of normal size. In addition, a large quantity of active substance and polymers requires the use of a large quantity of organic solvent.

There are at least theoretical solutions to these two problems. The large volume is less of a problem in dosage forms such as instant or effervescent granules of ibuprofen [505], while the use of large quantities of solvents can sometimes be avoided by using a solvent-free production process such as the roll-mixing process for triturations.

2.4.3.7
Further publications

In addition to the publications listed in Table 78 to 80, there is a series of further literature sources in which only the dissolution or the crystallinity of the solid solutions is investigated, without any determination of their stability, bioavailability or solubilization effect (i.e. increase in absolute solubility, see Section 2.4.5). Table 83 below gives an selection of such publications.

Table 83. Literature on solid solutions/dispersions with povidone, without stability, bioavailability or solubilization results (selection)

Acetylsalicylic acid [40 a, 40 b]
Albendazole [537]
Benidipine [147]
beta-Carotene [28, 42, 43]
Carbamazepine [252]
Chloramphenicol [44 b, 229]
Chlormadinone acetate [46]
Dexamethasone [59]
Diazepam [183]
Digoxin, Acetyldigoxin [105, 112, 204]
Dihydroergotamine [109, 263]
Dipyridamole [268]
Disopyramide [260]
Felodipine [531]
Furosemide [258]
Glibenclamide [237]
Gramicidin [49]
Griseofulvin [50, 161]
Hydrochlorothiazide [52 b]
Hydrocortisone [139, 148]
Ibuprofen [255]
Indomethacin [52 b, 152, 155, 195, 236]
Medazepam [31, 227]
Mefruside [219]
Methandrostenolone [52 b]
Methylprednisolone [52 b]
Nabilone [257]
Nalidixic acid [208]
Naproxen [264]
Nimodipine [577]
Nitrofurantoin [25]
Nystatin [56]
Oestradiol [57, 592, 629 melt extrusion]
Papaverine [200]
Piroxicam [585]

▶

Table 83. Continued

Prednisolone [437]
Prednisone [52b, 148]
Propylthiouracil [348]
Spironolactone [206]
Streptomycin sulphate [60]
Sulfamethoxazole [349]
Sulfaperine [54, 59]
Temazepan [597]
Terfenadine [470]
Tolazamide [199]
Tolbutamide [177]
Trimethoprim [153, 496]

2.4.4 Tablet coatings

2.4.4.1 *Sugar coating*

Mainly povidone K 25 and Kollidon 30 are used in sugar coating. The use of povidone K 90 often leads to an excessive increase in viscosity. Povidone K 25 and povidone K 30 have a number of physical properties (Table 84) that benefit the coating process and improve the quality of the coatings.

Sugar coatings are particularly susceptible to cracking when they are applied to large batches of tablet cores that are dried rapidly. As most active substances are hydrophobic, povidone K 25 and povidone K 30 are useful as additives to prevent the tablet coating cracking away from the tablet core during manufacture. Particularly when soluble dyes are used, povidone K 25 and povidone K 30 are useful in achieving an even distribution of the dye and preventing its migration, as well as increasing the capacity of the coating suspension for the dye.

When it is combined with small amounts of sodium dodecyl sulfate, povidone stabilizes suspensions of iron oxide pigment particles [421].

The formulation for a sugar-coating solution in Table 85 was taken from one of the many publications on the use of povidone in sugar coating [168–173].

Apart from its use in traditional manual sugar coating, povidone makes it possible to automate the sugar coating process. Table 86 gives a suitable formulation.

2.4.4.2 *Film coatings*

The properties given in Table 84 for povidone are also useful in the film-coating of tablets and hard gelatin capsules [281].

Table 84. Important properties and functions of povidone and copovidone for tablet coatings

Property	Function
Film formation	Avoidance of hairline cracks/crazing
Adhesion	Adhesion of the sugar layer to the tablet core
Affinity to hydrophobic surfaces	Adhesion of the tablet coating to cores with hydrophobic substances
Dispersive effect	Homogeneous distribution of the pigment or colour lake in the tablet coating
	Stabilization of the coating suspension
Retardation of crystallization	Slower and more homogeneous crystallization of the sugar

Table 85. Coating suspension with povidone for manual sugar coating

Sucrose	2130 g
Titanium dioxide	45 g
Povidone K 30	15 g
Colour lake	12 g
Poloxamer 188	3 g
Water	870 g

Table 86. Suspension for automatic sugar coating [231]

Sucrose	76 g
Povidone K 30	8 g
Titanium dioxide	9 g
Calcium carbonate	9 g
Talc	29 g
Colorant/pigment	q. s.
Glycerol	4 g
Water	63 g

40 kg of tablet cores with a weight of 420 mg were sprayed with 25 kg of the above suspension in a conventional coating pan under the following conditions:

Spray phase:	5 s
Interval:	10 min
Drying phase (warm air):	10 min
Total coating time:	16 h

The glass transition temperatures (Tg) of the different povidone types lie between 90°C and 189°C, depending on their molecular weight and on the moisture content [524]. Tg values of 130°C, 155°C, 168°C and 178°C have been measured for dried povidone K 17, povidone K 25, povidone K 30 and povidone K 90 [485].

Povidone K 90 is only seldom used for film coating (see Table 87). Its most important properties here are film formation, adhesion promotion [276], pigment dispersion and the improvement of the solubility of other film-forming agents and of the final coating in water [100].

A disadvantage of povidone in film-coating is its hygroscopicity (see Section 2.2.5). This is why they are normally never used as the sole film-forming agent for tablets. Table 87 gives formulations for coating solutions containing ethylcellulose and shellac, which give non-stick tablet coatings [176]. The incorporation of povidone in these soluble film coatings brings about an increase in the dissolution rate of the other film-forming agent, thus accelerating the disintegration of the tablet and the release of the active substance [100].

In formulations with shellac, povidone can be used to compensate for variations in quality of this natural product, which can affect the flexibility and dissolution rate of the coating [174, 175]. In other formulations, it may be possible to reduce the quantity of povidone (10–20%, in terms of the shellac) [174].

Table 87. Film-coating solutions with ethylcellulose or shellac and povidone [176]

	Shellac	Ethylcellulose
Povidone K 30	125 g	125 g
Povidone K 90	125 g	125 g
Shellac	250 g	–
Ethylcellulose 10 mPa s	–	250 g
Diethyl phthalate	200 g	200 g
Colorant	q. s.	q. s.
Ethanol 75%	ad 10 kg	ad 10 kg

Table 88. Enteric coating with methacrylic acid copolymer and povidone

I	Methacrylic acid copolymer dispersion 30 %, Ph.Eur.	100 g
	Water	200 g
II	Povidone K 25	6 g
	Propylene glycol	3 g
	Talc	45 g
	Titanium dioxide + pigments	35 g
	Silicone emulsion	1 g
	Water	210 g

Mix I and II and mill the suspension prior to use.

Povidone has also proved useful in polyacrylate film coatings. Table 88 gives a formulation for a spray suspension for enteric coatings.

2.4.4.3
Subcoatings for tablet cores

As mostly aqueous solutions and dispersions are used for coating these days, it has become increasingly necessary to provide the tablet cores with a subcoating before sugar or film-coating. This is mainly to provide a barrier to protect active substances in the tablet core that are sensitive to water, i.e. substances that are prone to hydrolysis or react with each other in the presence of water, e.g. vitamins, or to avoid swelling of high-performance tablet disintegrants, which start to swell even with small quantities of water. From Table 89 it can be seen that povidone is also able to hydrophilize the surface of the tablet core and reduce dust formation.

Subcoating with povidone K 30 is best carried out in the same machine as the subsequent sugar or film coating. Using a 10% solution of povidone K 30 in 2-propanol or ethanol, adequate protection can be obtained with a coating of less than 1 mg of povidone/cm^2 tablet surface.

Table 89. Reasons for subcoating tablet cores and the function of povidone and copovidone in these applications

Reasons for subcoating tablet cores	Function
Instability of the active substance towards water (hydrolysis)	Formation of a barrier layer on the surface and in the pores
Chemical reactions between the active substances (e.g. vitamins)	Formation of a barrier layer on the surface and in the pores
The presence of high-performance disintegrants	Formation of a barrier layer on the surface and in the pores
Hydrophobic surface of the tablet core	Improvement in adhesion of subsequent coatings by hydrophilization of the surface
Dust formation (friability of the tablet cores)	Loose particles are bound to the surface of the tablet core

2.4.5 Improvement of the solubility of drugs (solubilization)

2.4.5.1 *General*

As the majority of the active substances used today have relatively poor solubility in water, and organic solvents are very seldom used in liquid dosage forms, the use of auxiliaries for solubilization is playing an increasingly important role.

The excellent solubility in water of povidone as well as its ability to form water-soluble complexes with active substances can be taken advantage of to increase the absolute solubility of an active substance. As explained in Section 2.2.7, whether an active substance forms a complex with povidone depends on its chemical structure.

This property can be taken advantage of in almost all liquid dosage forms (Table 90), though in particular applications, some types of povidone are more suitable than others.

There is a direct connection between the use of povidone as a solubilizer and its function in delaying crystallization. This is particularly important in suspensions as recrystallization of the dissolved active substances brings about significant changes in the physical properties of the suspension (volume of sediment, redispersibility by shaking).

Table 90. Povidone used as solubilizers in liquid dosage forms

Dosage form	Povidone type 12	17	25	30	90
Injectables (solutions or suspensions)	+	+	–	–	–
Lyophilisates for injection	+	+	–	–	–
Lyophilisates for oral administration	–	–	+	+	+
Oral drops	–	–	+	+	+
Syrups, oral solutions	–	–	+	+	+
Ophthalmic products	–	+	+	+	+
Nose drops, ear drops	–	+	+	+	+
Topical solutions	–	–	+	+	+

2.4.5.2
Injectables for human and veterinary administration

When drugs are to be administered by the parenteral route, solubilization plays a more important role than in oral administration, as with the latter, a solid dosage form is equally acceptable. Therefore the endotoxin-free types, povidone K 12 and povidone K 17 are recommended for parenterals. The molecular weight of both products is low enough (see Section 2.2.6) to allow rapid renal elimination without storage. In many countries in Europe, e.g. Germany and Austria, only such low-molecular povidone types with a K-value of up to 18 are approved for injection (see Section 6.1.3).

Low-molecular povidones are nowadays widely used in different injectables e.g. in antibiotic and sulfonamide formulations. Fig. 54 shows, as an example, how the solubilization of rifampicin depends directly on the povidone concentration.

A similar linear relationship between the concentrations of povidone and solubilized active ingredient was found for sulindac [604].

In some veterinary injectables low molecular weight povidone is combined with 2-pyrrolidone. Typical examples are oxytetracycline [163], ivermectin [628] and sulfonamides [164].

Table 91 shows the composition of a commercially available oxytetracycline preparation for injection, that contains povidone as a solubilizing agent.

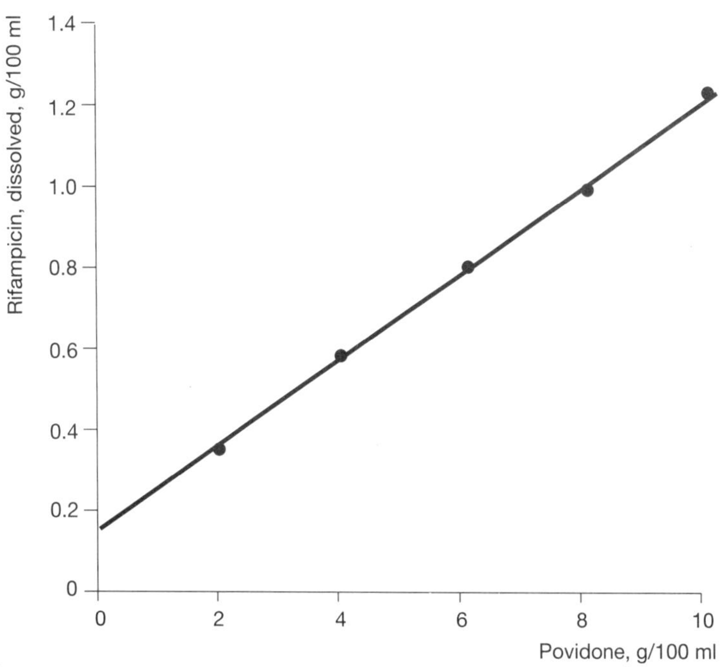

Fig. 54. Solubilization of rifampicin with low-molecular povidone [270]

Table 91. Composition of a commercially available oxytetracycline ampoule [113]

Oxytetracycline hydrochloride	5.70 g
Magnesium oxide	0.46 g
Reducing agent	0.50 g
Povidone K 17	10.00 g
Ethanolamine	q. s. (pH 8.8)
Water	ad 100 ml

Table 92. Influence of the molecular weight of the povidone type on solubilization

Povidone type	Active substance dissolved in 25% aqueous povidone solution	
	Trimethoprim	Phenobarbital
Without	0.4 mg/ml	ca. 1 mg/ml
Povidone K 12	2.5 mg/ml	10.5 mg/ml
Povidone K 17	5.0 mg/ml	12.5 mg/ml
Povidone K 25	10.0 mg/ml	>13 mg/ml

A positive side-effect of the use of povidone is a reduction in the local toxicity of oxytetracycline.

There are a large number of publications and papers in which the increase in absolute solubility of active substances by povidone has been tested and described. However, if the selection is restricted to the low-molecular types, this number becomes significantly smaller (Table 93). Naturally, a solubilization effect can also be expected of povidone K 12 and povidone K 17, even if such an effect is reported in the literature only for the medium-molecular povidone (see Table 97), though the amounts of active substance complexed may differ according to the molecular weight of povidone (see Table 92). However, the influence of the molecular weight depends very much on the active substance: with trimethoprim and chloramphenicol it is very large, while with phenobarbital it is small.

2.4.5.3
Lyophilisates

Lyophilisates are produced for parenteral and for oral preparations, e.g. drink ampoules. Povidone is used to bind the lyophilisate together during freeze-drying and to improve the solubility, stability and even the absorption of the active ingredient by virtue of its hydrophilic and complexing properties [185, 186, 244–249, 264, 278, 424, 482, 622, 656]. A typical example is melphalan [608, 611]. Table 94 shows a simple example of an antibiotic lyophilisate. An important reason for incorporating antibiotics in lyophilisates is that they are more stable in this form than in solutions.

Table 93. Solubilization of active substances through the use of low-molecular povidone grades (see also Table 97)

Active substance	Solubility increase factor	Ratio of drug to povidone	Literature source
Acetaminophen	1.2–2.3	1 + 9	[154, 659]
Acronycine	15–20	1 + 10	[200]
Ajmaline	ca. 10	1 + 5	[33]
Allopurinol	–	–	[32]
Amoxicillin	–	2 + 1–1 + 3	[185]
Carbamazepine	–	–	[529]
Chloramphenicol	>15	1 + 10	–
Clonazepam	16	–	[149 b]
Danofloxacin	–	1 + 1	[626]
Doxycycline	–	–	[110]
Flunitrazepam	9	–	[149 b]
Furaltadone	ca. 7	1 + 5	–
Hydrochlorothiazide	7–9	1 + 4	[53, 550]
Hydroflumethiazide	4	3 + 1	[34, 316]
Hydroxystaurosprine	500	–	[552]
Metronidazole	5	1 + 5	–
Nitrazepam	13	–	[149 b]
Oxytetracycline	>13	1 + 1	[22, 23, 163, 193, 562]
Piroxicam	–	1 + 2	[512]
Prednisolone	2	1 + 10	[345]
Rafoxanide	–	1 + 3	[182]
Rifampicin	> 6	1 + 6	[270]
Sulfadimethoxine	–	–	[164]
Sulfamethazine	–	–	[164]
Sulfamoxole	–	–	[21]
Sulfathiazole	3–4	1 + 1–1 + 20	[30 a + 30 c]
Tenidap	> 30	3 + 1	[526]
Trimethoprim	>12	1 + 50	[496]

Table 94. Amoxicillin lyophilisate for injection [185]

Amoxicillin sodium	6.25 g
Povidone K 12	7.50 g
Water for injections	ad 100 ml

After freeze-drying, fill 550-mg portions of the lyophilisate into ampoules.

Prior to administration, the contents of an ampoule are mixed with 1.9 ml of water to give a clear injection solution.

2.4.5.4
Oral and topical solutions

Povidone can be used in oral drops, oral solutions, syrups and in topical solutions to improve the solubility of active substances in the same way as in parenteral dosage forms. The medium and higher molecular weight grades, are usually used for this purpose, as they increase the viscosity of the solutions, which can be an advantage in providing a constant drip rate or improving the appearance or the adhesion to the skin.

Tables 95 and 96 give formulations for acetaminophen and diclofenac oral solutions that were developed on a laboratory scale, as typical examples. In the case of acetaminophen, povidone not only solubilizes the active substance, it also reduces its bitter taste [625]. Similar effects are described in the case of sulfamethoxazol and trimethoprim [21, 625].

Further to the active substances listed in Table 93, that can be solubilized with the low-molecular grades of povidone, Table 97 gives a series of further active substances whose solubility can be increased with medium and high-molecular povidone. Naturally, the solubility of the active substances listed in Table 93 can also be improved with povidone K 25, povidone K 30 or povidone K 90, though not always to the same extent (Table 92).

Table 95. Acetaminophen oral solution (500 mg/10 ml)

Acetaminophen (paracetamol)	50 g
Sorbitol, cryst.	50 g
Povidone K 25	200 g
Sodium cyclamate	30 g
Propylene glycol	200 g
Flavouring	2 g
Glycerol	150 g
Water	318 g

Dissolve all the solid substances in a mixture of the liquid components at room temperature.

Table 96. Diclofenac oral solution (1.5 %)

Diclofenac sodium	1.5 g
Povidone K 30	2.5 g
Sucrose	40.0 g
Water	56.0 g

Dissolve povidone and then diclofenac sodium in the sucrose syrup.

Table 97. Further active substances whose solubility can be increased with povidone (supplement to Table 93)

Active substance	Solubility increase factor (where given)	Ratio of drug to povidone (where given)	Literature source
Acronycine	15	1 + 5	[41]
alpha-Asarone	> 40	1 + 10	[329]
Aminobenzoic acid		1 + 1	[269]
Armillarisine	6	1 + 5	[331]
Carmofur	6	1 + 5	[332]
Chloramphenicol	1.3	1 + 1	[228]
Chlordiazepoxide	1.7–3.5	1 + 25	[104, 228, 254]
Chlorhexidine			[356]
Chlorpropamide	5		[266]
Cinnarizine	2	1 + 3	[165, 333]
Cloxacillin			[334]
Coumarin		2 + 3	[25]
Dapsone			[356]
Diazepam	2	1 + 25	[254]
Diclofenac		1 + 3	[630]
Dicumarol	> 20		[35]
Diethylstilbestrol	1.5–2		[151, 188]
Drotaverine	1.8	1 + 2	[48]
Emodin			[336]
Ergot alkaloids			[337]
Erythromycin		1 + 5	[242, 338]
Ethotoin		1 + 8	[25]
Furosemide			[356]
Glibenclamide			[339]
Gramicidin		1 + 3	[49]
Griseofulvin	2	1 +	[24, 337, 340]
Hydroflumethiazide	4	1 + 3	[341]
Ibuprofen	8	1 + 1	[277, 342]
Indomethacin			[333, 356]
Ketoprofen		1 + 2	[196]
Lonetil	2	1 + 10	[136, 333]
Lorazepam			[330]
Medazepam		1 + 25	[104, 254]
Nifedipine	3.5	1 + 3	[205]
Nitrofural	4		[162]
Nitrofurantoin	3–5		[162]
Nystatin	6–10	1 + 5	[52 b, 301, 343, 347]
Oxazepam			[228]
Pentazocine napsylate	> 8	1 + 3	[344]
Phenobarbital	2	1 + 10	[159]
Phenytoin	1.5	1 + 10	[187, 256, 326]
Prednisolone	2–4		[26, 162]

▶

Table 97. Continued

Active substance	Solubility increase factor (where given)	Ratio of drug to povidone (where given)	Literature source
Progesterone	2.8		[151]
Quercetin			[334]
Reserpine	3.5	1 + 10	[27, 305]
Rutin			[334]
Spironolactone			[346]
Sulfathiazole	10	1 + 2	[138]
Sulindac	4		[604]
Testosterone	2		[151]
Tetramisole	–	2 + 1	[579]
Tranilast		1 + 3	[354, 596]
Tyrothricin	–	1 + 2	[29, 49]

2.4.5.5
Ophthalmic solutions

The ability of povidone to increase the solubility of active substances is just as useful in eye drops as in parenterals (Table 98).

Table 99 below gives an example of a formulation for a 3% chloramphenicol solution developed on a laboratory scale for application to the eye.

The film-forming and viscosity-increasing effects of the povidone have been recognized as positive side-effects in ophthalmic solutions (see Section 2.4.7).

Table 98. Examples of active substances for ophthalmic preparations, that can be solubilized with povidone

Chloramphenicol
Prednisolone
Rifampicin
Tyrothricin

Table 99. Chloramphenicol solution for eye drops [615]

Chloramphenicol	3.0 g
Povidone K 25	15.0 g
Preservative	q.s.
Water	ad 100.0 g

2.4.5.6
Soft gelatin capsules

To obtain clear soft gelatin capsules of insoluble drug substances povidone and e.g. triesters of citric acid can be combined [560].

2.4.6
Suspensions, dry syrups and instant granules

2.4.6.1
General

Various auxiliaries with different functions are used in suspensions or dry syrups and instant granules for the preparation of suspensions. These include thickeners, hydrophilic polymers as dispersing agents, sugars, surfactants, electrolytes, colorants, etc. [296].

All povidone types can be used as hydrophilic polymers to physically stabilize suspensions [39, 119]. Their most important and primary function in all suspensions is as protective colloids, which hydrophilize the individual solid particles and sterically separate them. This increases the volume of any sediment and makes it easier to redisperse by shaking. Povidone also prevents the dissolved portion of the active substance from crystallizing out by forming soluble complexes with it [389] (see also Sections 2.2.7 and 2.4.5). The Zeta potential of many substances, e. g. iron oxide pigments, can also be reduced with povidone [421].

2.4.6.2
Oral suspensions, dry syrups and instant granules

In addition to the functions given above, the thickening effect of povidone is also used in oral suspensions. This particularly applies to povidone K 90, which gives solutions of significantly higher viscosity than, for example, povidone K 25 (Section 2.2.3). The effect of the viscosity on the sedimentation rate of a suspension is given by Stokes' Law for Newtonian fluids:

$$\text{Sedimentation rate} = \frac{2\,r^2\,(d1 - d2)g}{9\,\eta} \quad (\text{cm/s})$$

η = Viscosity of the suspension
r = Radius of the particles
d1 = Density of the suspended phase
d2 = Density of the continuous phase
g = Gravity

If the suspension has pseudoplastic properties, the sedimentation rate is greater according to the difference between the gravitational force on the suspended particles and the yield point of the system. Thus the sedimentation rate of such systems can also be reduced by a thickening agent such as povidone K 90.

With some suspensions it was actually found that the sediment volume was directly proportional to the viscosity over a certain range, which confirms that Stokes' Law can be applied here [370].

Figure 55 shows the influence of an addition povidone K 90 on the sedimentation behaviour of micronized crospovidone in water at different concentrations. A 7.5% suspension of micronized crospovidone to which 5% povidone K 90 had been added showed no sedimentation within 24 hours, and its redispersibility was very good. Without povidone, significant amounts of crospovidone settled out.

The active substances that are most frequently marketed in the form of suspensions or dry syrups and instant granules for the preparation of suspensions are antibiotics, chemotherapeutics and antiacids. Table 100 gives a formulation that was developed in the laboratory for an antacid suspension with povidone K 90.

Further examples of laboratory formulations for dry syrups, instant granules and suspensions are given in Section 3.4.4.3.

In granules for the preparation of suspensions, povidone can also act as a binder (see Table 75).

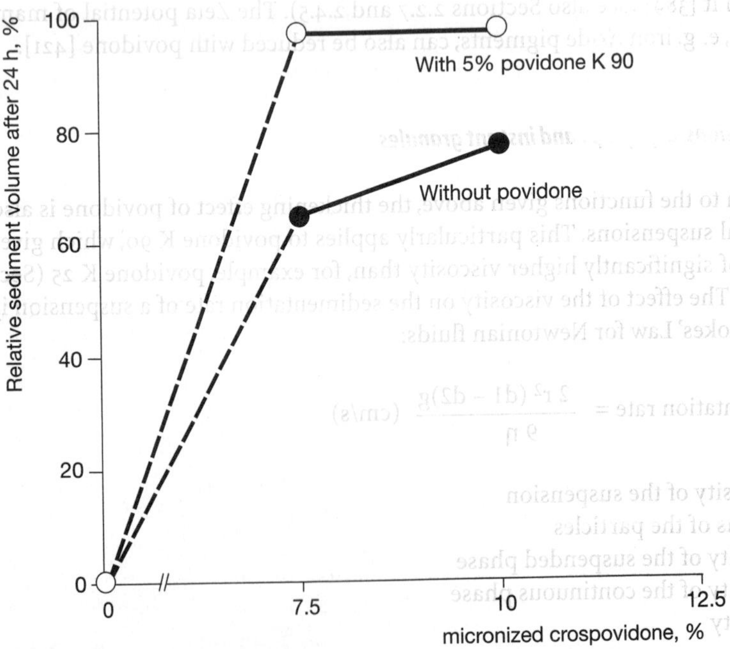

Fig. 55. Reduction in sedimentation of micronized crospovidone (low bulk density) with povidone K 90

Table 100. Magaldrate antiacid suspension

Magaldrate (USP)	100.0 g
Micromized crospovidone (low bulk density)	80.0 g
Povidone K 90	30.0 g
Sucrose	150.0 g
Orange flavouring	9.0 g
Coconut flavouring	0.5 g
Banana flavouring	0.8 g
Saccharin sodium	0.2 g
(Preservative	q. s.)
Water	ad 1000.0 ml

Dissolve or suspend all the solids in water under aseptic conditions.

Properties of the suspension:
- Remains homogeneous without sedimentation for more than 24 hours.
- Very readily redispersed after 2 weeks by shaking.

The use of the povidone in sugar-coating suspensions is described in Section 2.4.4 and their use in ophthalmic suspensions in Section 2.4.7.

2.4.6.3 Parenteral suspensions

Low-molecular povidones can be used as dispersing agents for parenteral suspensions (crystalline suspensions, lyophilisates, nanoparticles) [115, 116, 120–122, 633]. These endotoxin-free grades have been developed specially for parenterals and produce suspensions with about the same physical properties as, for example, povidone K 30, except that their viscosity is somewhat lower.

Some typical active ingredients combined with low molecular weight povidone in commercialized parenteral suspensions are benzylpenicillin, fluspirilen, penicillin and streptomycin.

2.4.7 Applications in ophthalmic solutions

All povidone types have applications in ophthalmic solutions [83–86, 102, 267, 354]. Povidone K 17, povidone K 25 and povidone K 30 are usually used in eye drops while the higher-molecular type, povidone K 90, is preferred for contact lens solutions [87, 88, 203, 382]. It is usually added to these dosage forms in concentrations between 2% and 10% and performs the functions shown in Table 101.

The *film formation* and *thickening* actions of povidone, and sometimes also its ability to form complexes with active ingredients, keep the solution in the eye for a longer time, increasing its therapeutic effect. Pilocarpine [86], timolol [166] and

Table 101. Functions of povidone in ophthalmic solutions

- Film formation
- Thickening (see Sections 2.2.3 and 2.4.8.1)
- Prolonged retention of the active substance in the eye
- Increase in bioavailability (see Section 2.4.3)
- Lubrication (Dry eye syndrom) [623, 624]
- Solubilization of active substances (see Section 2.4.5)
- Reduction of eye irritation caused by some active substances

Table 102. Sodium perborate effervescent tablet for cleaning contact lenses [382]

Sodium perborate	69.2
Sodium hydrogen carbonate	260.0
EDTA sodium	27.4
Citric acid	121.6
Povidone K 30	4.6
Polyethylene glycol 6000	9.2
EDTA manganese	8.0

tropicamide [442] are two typical active ingredients whose efficacy can be improved by these properties. Both properties also increase the lubricant effect, e.g. in tear fluid substitute [558].

The general *improvement in bioavailability* of active substances that is brought about by povidone is described in Section 2.4.3. However, there are also a number of publications that investigate this parameter specifically in ophthalmic preparations [230, 235, 267, 427, 442, 480] or ocular delivery systems of fluorometholone [598].

The *solubilization* of active substances, such as chloramphenicol, in eye drops is described in Section 2.4.5.5, Table 99.

Oxymetazoline is a typical example of a substance, whose *irritation effect on the eye can be reduced* by soluble povidone.

Povidone can also be used as a sedimentation stabilizer in ophthalmic suspensions. Mefenamic acid suspension is a typical example [492].

The use of povidone K 30 in effervescent cleaning tablets for contact lenses is an indirect ophthalmic application. Table 102 shows the composition of a perborate cleaning tablet taken from the literature.

2.4.8
Sustained-release preparations

2.4.8.1
General informations

Because of its excellent solubility, povidone normally have no delaying effect on the dissolution of active substances. Though a substance embedded in povidone K 90 dissolves slightly more slowly than it would in povidone K 30, this minor difference cannot be described as a controlled-release effect. On the contrary, the dissolution rate is frequently higher than that of the pure drug (see Sections 2.4.3 and 2.4.5). However, in the case of papaverine tablets, a pH-independent sustained release was found [495].

A number of publications appeared since 1981, in which it was reported that povidone forms insoluble flocculates with polyacrylic acid and that these can be used to control release by enveloping crystals or tablet cores in the flocculate [407–410, 520, 583].

Povidone can also be used as a hydrophilic component or pore former in preparations that contain sustained-release auxiliaries like polyvinyl acetate, cellulose derivatives like HPMC [490, 509, 660], alginate [461], cetylacohol [600], polylactic acid [506], Gelucire®* [510], polyvinyl alcohol [522], ceresine wax [523], stearic acid [606] or methacrylate copolymers [491] to control or regulate the release of active substances, as binders and/or sometimes as plasticizers. They can also be extruded together with the active substance in melted stearyl alcohol and filled into hard gelatin capsules to achieve the same effect [471]. Ocular delivery systems are also described [598].

2.4.8.2
Spray-dried polyvinyl acetate/povidone mixture 8+2

Recently a spray-dried mixture of 8 parts of polyvinyl acetate (PVAc) and 2 parts of povidone K 30 can be found in the market. It is recommended as matrix for sustained-release tablets obtained by direct compression. In this product povidone has two functions: to get a free-flowing polyvinyl acetate powder and to form pores in the tablets.

The spray dried PVAc/Povidone powder offers outstanding flow properties having a response angle well below 30°. It can enhance the flowability of other components added for a tablet formulation of direct compression. Figure 56 illustrates its flowability as one of the main justifications for the use in the direct compression technology in comparison to other sustained-release matrix formers of the market. The angle of repose of the other substances is significantly higher than the usual limit of 32 to 33°. Therefore they are used almost only in the wet granulation technology of tablets.

* Gelucire® is a registered trademark of Gattefossé SA, Saint Priest, France

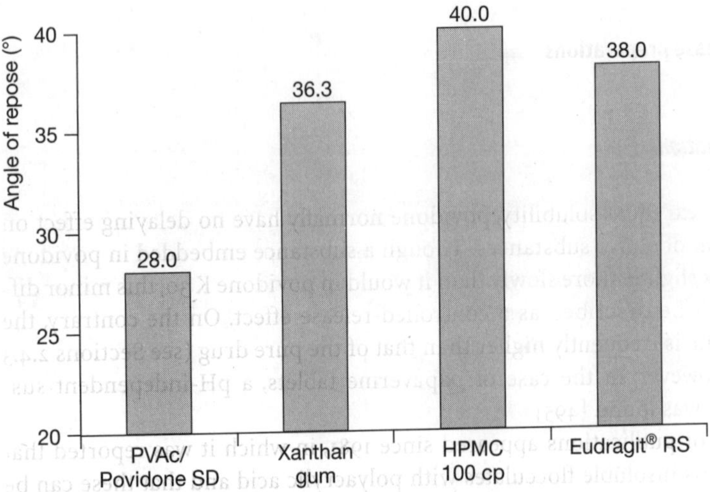

Fig. 56. Flowability of spray-dried PVAc/Povidone in comparison with some other sustained-release matrix formers

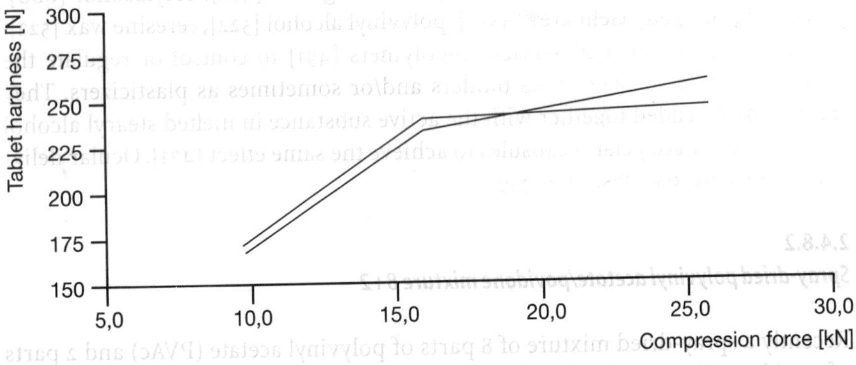

Fig. 57. Compressibility of two batches of spray-dried PVAc/Povidone in propranolol tablets (Formulation see Table 104)

The high compressibility as an expression of the excellent dry binding properties is an other important parameter for the use in the direct compression technology of tablets. Figure 57 shows the extremely high tablet hardness levels obtained with different compression forces on propranolol tablets. This is due the combination of the very plastic polyvinyl acetate and the strongly binding povidone.

2.4.8.3
Applications of spray-dried PVAc/Povidone 8:2 as sustained-release matrix

Spray-dried PVAc/Povidone can be used for the production of sustained-release matrix tablets and pellets.

Different technologies to obtain such dosage forms can be applied: Direct compression, roller compaction, melt extrusion and wet granulation. In the case of the wet granulation PVAc/Povidone should be added to the extragranular phase.

The excellent flowability and compressibility of spray-dried PVAc/Povidone makes this excipient particulary suitable for the manufacture of sustained-release tablets obtained by *direct compression* [647–649].

The required concentration in the tablet depends mainly on the particle size and the solubility of the active ingredient. The finer the particles the faster is the dissolution. Table 103 gives an information about the usual amounts to obtain a sustained release during 12–24 hours.

The sustained-release characteristics can be modified by varying the content of spray-dried PVAc/Povidone in the formulation. Figure 58 shows the influence of the amount of on the release of caffeine as a example of a soluble active ingredient.

Tables 103. Usual amounts of spray-dried PVAc/Povidone in tablets

Solubility of the active ingredient	Amount in the tablet
Very slightly soluble to practically insoluble	15–25%
Sparingly soluble to slightly soluble	25–40%
Soluble to freely soluble	40–55%

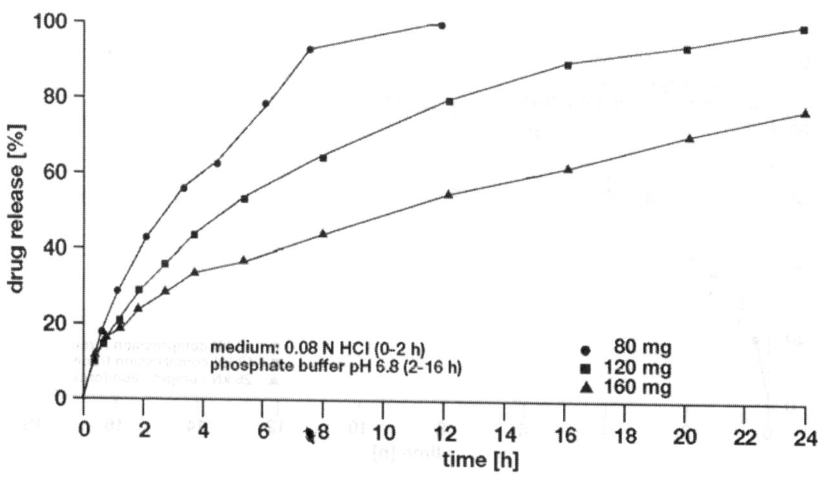

Fig. 58. Influence of the amount of spray-dried PVAc/Povidone on the drug release in caffeine sustained-release tablet (160 mg caffeine)

In the case of slightly soluble or practically insoluble drug substances the release can be accelerated not only by reducing the content of PVAc/Povidone but also by the addition of hydrophilic substances like (granulated) lactose, povidone K 30 or micronized crospovidone which act as pore former.

Outstanding and important properties of sustained release matrix tablets based on PVAc/Povidone are the following:

1. The drug release is independent of the pH (see Fig. 59).
2. The drug release is independent of the ionic strength of the dissolution medium (see Fig. 59, addition of 2.5% of NaCl).
3. The drug release is independent of the usual compression force and tablet hardness (see Fig. 60).

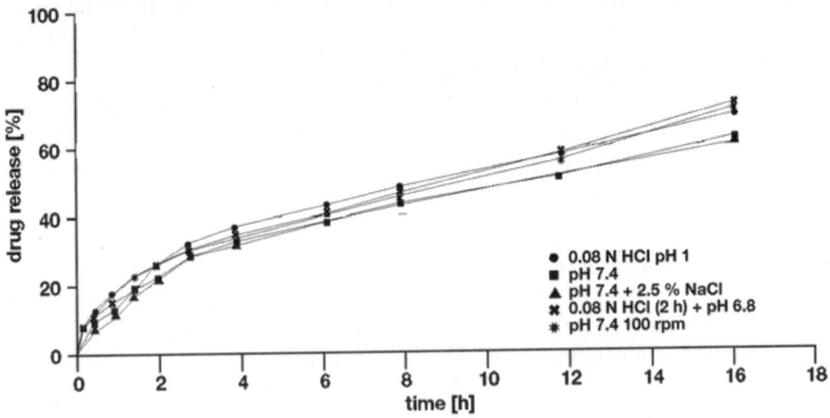

Fig. 59. Influence of the pH and the ionic strength of the dissolution medium on the release of caffeine tablets (Caffeine + spray-dried PVAc/Povidone 1+1)

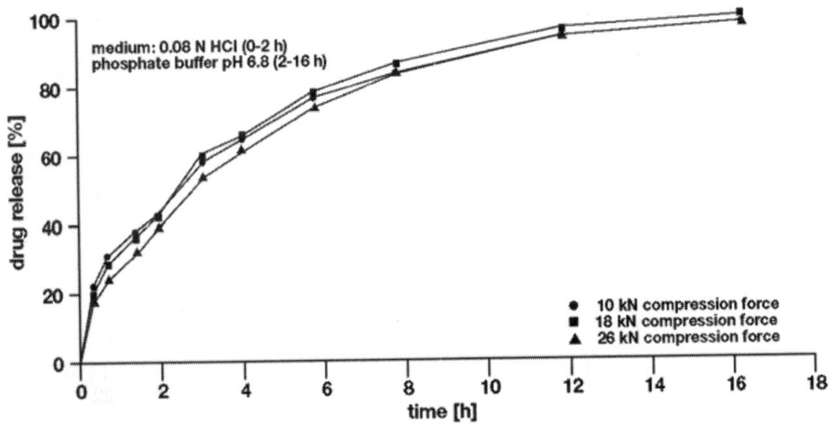

Fig. 60. Propranolol sustained-release tablets: Influence of the compression force on the drug release

It is recommended to store the matrix tablets at temperatures below 30°C and in tightly closed containers to avoid the uptake of humidity which could modify the release profile of formulations.

2.4.8.4
Sustained-release formulations with spray-dried PVAc/Povidone 8:2

For the production of sustained-release tablets with spray-dried PVAc/povidone as matrix the direct compression technology is recommended.

In the Tables 104 to 105 typical examples of soluble and practically insoluble active ingredients are given in form of sustained-release tablets. Further formulations can be found in the literature [615].

If the wet granulation technology is applied spray-dried PVAc/Povidone should be put in the extragranular phase to avoid the wetting of this polymer mixture. Such application is shown in in Table 106 in a formulation of metoprolol sustained-release tablets.

Polyvinyl acetate is described in the literature as a matrix former in theophylline sustained-release tablets obtained by hot-melt extrusion [646]. In a similar way spray-dried PVAc/Povidone can be applied for the production of tablets and pellets using its excellent flowability. In this case the pulverization of polyvinyl acetate by cryogenic grinding can be avoided and the mixture of the active ingredient with the excipients are applied directly to the melt extruder.

Table 104. Propranolol sustained-release tablets (160 mg)

	Parts by weight [g]	Composition [%]
Propranolol-HCl	160.0	49.23
Spray-dried PVAc/Povidone	160.0	49.23
Silicon dioxide, colloidal	3.4	1.05
Magnesium stearate	1.6	0.49
Total	325.0	100.00

Manufacture

All ingredients were passed through a 0.8 mm sieve, blended for 10 min in a Turbula mixer and then pressed to tablets on a rotary press.

Tablets properties

Diameter	10 mm
Weight	330 mg
Compression force	10 kN / 18 kN / 25 kN
Hardness	170 N / 235 N / 250 N
Friability	0.1 %
Drug release	See Fig. 60

Table 105. Theophylline sustained-release tablets (500 mg)

	Parts by weight [g]	Composition [%]
Theophylline gran. (BASF)	500.0	53.9
Spray-dried PVAc/Povidone	200.0	21.6
Granulated lactose	225.0	24.2
Magnesium stearate	3.0	0.3
Total	928.0	100.00

Manufacture
All ingredients were passed through a 0.8 mm sieve, blended for 10 min in a Turbula mixer and then pressed on a rotary press.

Tablet properties	
Diameter	19.0 x 8.5 mm (football shape)
Weight	928 mg
Compression force	11 kN
Hardness	172 N
Friability	< 0.1%
Drug release	See Figure 61

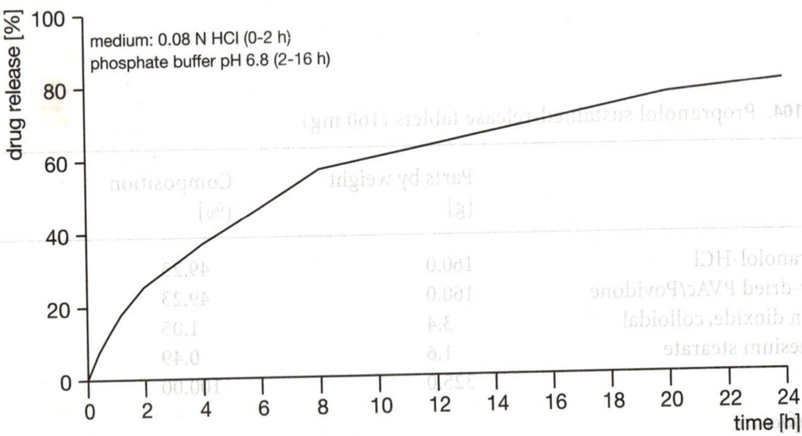

Fig. 61. Dissolution of theophylline sustained-release tablets

Table 106. Metoprolol sustained-release tablets (200 mg)

Formulation

I	Metoprolol tartrate (Moehs, Spain)	200 g
II	Polyvinyl acetate dispersion 30 %	20 g
III	Spray-dried PVAc/Povidone	250 g
	Magnesium stearate	2.5 g

Manufacture (Wet granulation)

Granulate substance I in a top spray fluidized bed with dispersion II (Inlet air temperature 50 °C, outlet air temperature about 26 °C, nozzle 1.2 mm), mix with III and press to tablets with low compression force (9 kN) on a rotary press.

Tablet properties

Diameter	12 mm
Weight	459 mg
Form	biplanar
Hardness	220 N
Friability	< 0.1%
Drug release	See Figure 62

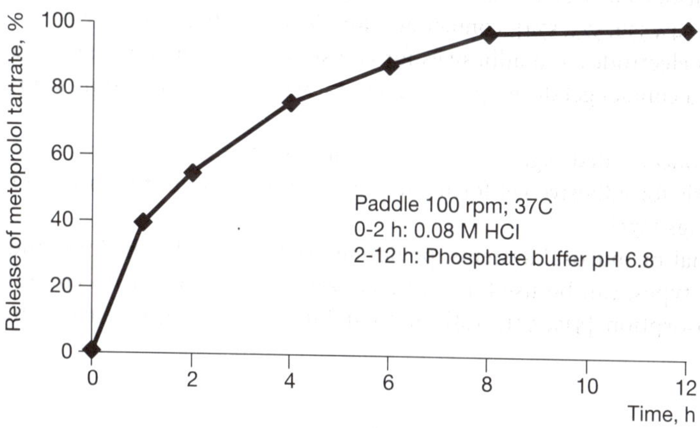

Fig. 62. Dissolution of metoprolol sustained-release tablets

2.4.9
Miscellaneous applications

2.4.9.1
Thickener for solutions

The medium-molecular povidones and above all the high-molecular grade, povidone K 90 are used as thickeners in oral and topical solutions and suspensions (viscosity curves, see Section 2.2.3). The use of povidone in suspensions is described in Section 2.4.6. The thickening effect can also be used to adjust the viscosity of solutions – oral drops, eye drops, solutions and syrups – to give a particular drip or flow rate. The thickening effect reduces diffusion processes in the solution, improving the stability of some active substances.

The good solubility of povidone in different solvents enables them to be used also as thickeners in aqueous/alcoholic preparations.

2.4.9.2
Adhesive gels, transdermal and mucosal systems

Because of their excellent adhesion and physiological safety, povidone K 30 and povidone K 90 are used as adhesives on the skin or mucous membranes. Examples include transdermal systems, oral adhesive gels, buccal adhesive patches or tablets [511, 546, 547, 559, 573, 574], contact gels for electrocardiograph or electroencephalograph electrodes and adhesives for colostomy bags. Table 107 shows a formulation for a contact gel developed on a laboratory scale for ultrasonic scanning.

A relatively concentrated, e.g. 20–30%, clear solution of povidone K 90 is adequate as the basis for adhesive gel formulations for application in the mouth or for colostomy bags [375].

In transdermal or mucosal systems, povidone, particularly the medium and high-molecular types, can be used as an bioadhesive, to improve or to control transdermal absorption [535, 571, 658], or to stabilize active ingredients or to

Table 107. Formulation for an ultrasonic contact gel

I	Povidone K 30	1.5 g
	Water	20.0 g
II	Preservative	0.5 g
	Carbopol®* 940	0.6 g
	Water	75.4 g
III	Sodium hydroxide solution 10% in water	2.0 g

Prepare Suspension II then add III and mix with Solution I.

* Carbopol® is a registered trademark of Noveon IP Holdings Corp., Cleveland, Ohio, USA

inhibit the crystallization of the drug [58]. The most important substances used in transdermal or mucosal systems, with which povidone can be used, include bromhexine [455], captopril [582], chlorhexidine [594], diclofenac [491], dilthiazem [599], ephedrine [417], flurbiprofen [627], hormone [559], hydrocortisone [412], indomethacin [599], isosorbide dinitrate [418, 518, 535, 570, 578], nabulphine [658], nitroglycerin [384-386, 578], pentazocine [539], promethazine [456], propranolol [578], salicylic acid [413, 415, 416], terbutalin [657], testosteron [514], tetracycline [632] and verapamil [563, 571] (see also Section 2.4.3.4).

2.4.9.3
Plastics for medical use

Many plastics materials are too hydrophobic for use in direct contact with body fluids such as blood, plasma, etc. Plastics are nowadays hydrophilized by different methods with povidone, e.g. povidone K 30 or povidone K 90 (Table 108) [494, 621].

By adding povidone during the polymerization of plastics, it is possible to adjust the size of the pores in the plastics material, used for filtration and dialysis purposes.

With the methods given in Table 108, great care must be taken that no high-molecular povidone can be leached out of or peeled away from the plastics material in the body or in contact with body fluids. Povidone K 90 and povidone K 30 become insoluble hydrophilic substances after crosslinking. Alkaline treatment, e.g. with sodium hydroxide is an established and effective method.

2.4.9.4
Reduction of the toxicity of active ingredients and other substances

Because of its ability to form complexes with a large number of substances (see Sections 2.2.7, 2.4.3 and 2.4.5) povidone can be used to reduce the toxicity of certain active substances (Table 109). This effect is mainly used with active substances such as oxytetracycline, that are given parenterally as well as those that are applied topically to the skin and to the eye (e.g. iodine, oxymetazoline).

Not only can the toxicity of active substances be reduced by povidone. The irritant or toxic effects of other substances such as cyanides, nicotine, formaldehyde, formamide, and other toxins, with which povidone forms complexes of adequate stability, can also be reduced [126].

Table 108. Applications of povidone in medical plastics

- Addition of povidone during polymerization of plastics (formation of pores)
- Coating of plastics with povidone followed by crosslinking by means of:
  1. Alkaline treatment [1, 141, 217]
  2. Radiation curing [371]
  3. Reaction with isocyanates and curing [621]

Table 109. Examples of pharmaceutical active substances whose reduction in toxicity by complexation with povidone is described in the literature

Active substance	Administration				Literature
	Parenteral	Topical	Ocular	Oral	
Acetylsalicylic acid	–	–	–	+	[189]
Azapropazone	–	–	–	+	[284, 319]
Closantel	+	–	–	–	
Floctafenine	–	–	–	+	[284, 319]
Florifenine	–	+	–	–	[545]
Glafenine	–	–	–	+	[284, 319]
Indomethacin	–	–	–	+	[123]
Iodine	–	+	(+)	–	[124]
Mefenamic acid	–	–	–	+	[284, 319]
Oxymetazoline	–	–	+	–	
Oxytetracycline	+	–	–	–	[22, 373, 374]
Polymyxin B	+	–	–	+	[489]
Temafloxacin	+	–	–	–	[517]

2.4.9.5
Cryoprotection

The inhibition of the crystallization of water and active substances by povidone has been investigated in a number of publications with respect to the freeze-drying of histological specimens. This cryoprotective effect therefore plays a greater role in biotechnology than in the manufacture of drugs (see also Section 2.4.5.3).

2.4.9.6
Stabilization of enzymes

Povidone, particularly the medium-molecular type, can be used to stabilize many enzymes, as is extensively described in the literature. Complexation also plays a role here in binding deactivating substances such as phenols and tannins. This and other properties are used to advantage both in diagnostic reagents, including those in the rapid test kits, and in microbiological processes. Table 110 contains a list of enzymes that, according to the literature, can be stabilized directly or indirectly by complexation with povidone.

2.4.9.7
Stabilization of active ingredients

Povidone is capable of chemically stabilizing certain active ingredients. This effect does not depend on the dosage form, as povidone is used to stabilize nitroglycerin and isosorbide dinitrate, particularly in transdermal systems [384–386],

Table 110. Stabilization of enzymes with povidone (selection)

Asparaginase
beta-Interferon
Catalase
Dehydrogenase
Ferrochelatase
Galactosidase
Glucose oxidase
Hyaluronidase
Peroxidase
Phenolase
Prostaglandin E
Pyruvate carboxilase
Transaminase
Urease

Table 111. Vitamin B complex parenteral solution [368d]

1. Formulation

I	Thiamine hydrochloride	11.0 mg
	Riboflavin monophosphate sodium	6.6 mg
	Nicotinamide	44.0 mg
	Pyridoxine hydrochloride	4.4 mg
	Cyanocobalamin	8.8 µg
	EDTA sodium	0.2 mg
	Propyl gallate	0.5 mg
	Povidone K 17	99.0 mg
II	Parabens	1.6 mg
	Citric acid	22.7 mg
	Sodium hydroxide solution, 1 mol/l	0.216 ml
	Hydrochloric acid, 0.1 mol/l	0.720 ml
	Propylene glycol	0.200 ml
	Water	0.864 ml

Dissolve Mixture I in Solution II, purge with nitrogen for 5 min, sterilize by filtration and fill into ampoules under nitrogen. The pH is about 4.

2. Stability (9 months, room temperature)

Vitamin	Loss
B_1	8 %
B_2	6 %
B_6	9 %
Nicotinamide	0 %
B_{12}	13 %

Table 112. Stabilization of active ingredients with povidone

Active ingredients	Literature
Ascorbic acid	[420]
Colecalciferol	[309]
Dehydroandrosteron sulfate	[424]
Erythrocytes	[507]
Hydrogen peroxide	[516]
Hydroxystaurosprine	[552]
Immunoglobulin	[515]
Interferon	[482]
Iodine	
Isosorbide dinitrate	
Methylprednisolone	[12]
Nitroglycerin	[422, 423]
Prostaglandin	[327]
Taurolidine	[568]
Theophylline	[569]
Thiamine hydrochloride	[419]
L-Tyroxin	[532]

iodine in topical solutions and vitamins in oral and parenteral solutions and in solid forms. Table 111 shows a formulation for a Vitamin B complex solution for parenterals, developed in the laboratory, in which the cyanocobalamin was found to be very unstable without the addition of povidone. The use of povidone K 17 reduced the loss of cyanocobalamin to only 13% during 9 months' storage.

Further active substances, in addition to cyanocobalamin, that can be stabilized povidone, are shown in Table 112.

2.4.9.9
Buccal preparations

Povidone reduces the adherence of oral bacteria to tooth enamel and therefore it could be used in buccal preparations e.g. mouthwash solution as microbial anti-adherent agent [589]. It also can be used as mucoadhesive for buccal coats of verapamil [612] or for bioadhesive buccal tablets of nicotine [639, 641].

3 Insoluble polyvinylpyrrolidone (Crospovidone)

3.1 Structure, product range, synonyms

Insoluble polyvinylpyrrolidone (crospovidone) is manufactured by a polymerization process that produces a mainly physically crosslinked popcorn polymer [2].

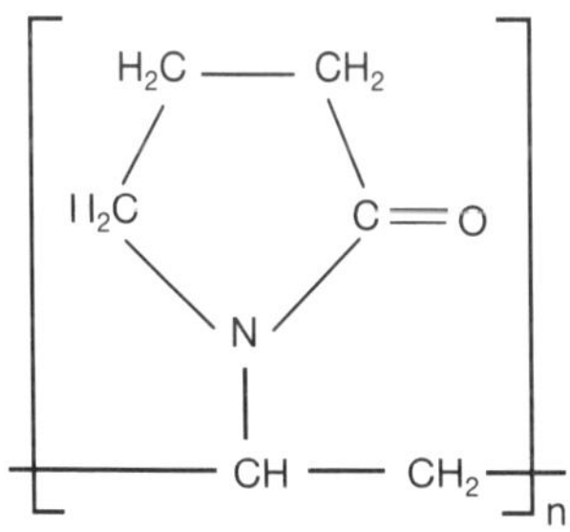

$Mr = (111.1)_x$

With crospovidone, it is not possible to use the molecular weight or the K-value as a means of identifying the different types, as is done with povidone, since crospovidone is completely insoluble and its molecular weight cannot be determined. Table 113 gives the product range available in the market.

Table 113. Crospovidone grades available in the market

Product (Trade name)	Manufacturer
Normal grades:	
Kollidon® CL	BASF
Polyplasdone®* XL	ISP
Micronized/fine powder grades:	
Kollidon® CL-M	BASF
Polyplasdone® XL-10	ISP
Polyplasdone® INF-10	ISP

* Polyplasdone® is a registered trademark of ISP Investments Inc., Wilmington, Delaware, USA

Table 114. General names and abbreviations for insoluble polyvinylpyrrolidone

Name/abbreviation	Origin/area of application
Crospovidone	Pharmacopoeias (e.g. USP, Ph.Eur.)
Crospovidonum	Ph. Eur.
Crospolyvidone	First Ph.Eur. draft 1991
Insoluble polyvidone	DAC until 1986
Insoluble PVP	General abbreviation
Crosslinked PVP	General abbreviation
Polyvinylpolypyrrolidone	Chemically incorrect designation often encountered in the food literature
PVPP	Abbreviation used in the beverages industry

The products differ in their physical properties, particularly in their bulk density, swelling characteristics and particle size (see Sections 3.2.2.1 to 3.2.2.3).

Insoluble polyvinylpyrrolidone has got the same CAS-number as soluble polyvinylpyrrolidone: 9003-39-8.

The names and abbreviations in Table 114 are generally used for insoluble polyvinylpyrrolidone in pharmaceuticals.

The designation polyvinylpolypyrrolidone (PVPP) is still used in the literature, although it is certainly not correct. This is confirmed by a comparison of the infrared spectra for crospovidone and povidone, which reveals no recognizable difference (see Section 3.3.1.1).

In the following sections of this chapter, only the term "crospovidone" is used for insoluble polyvinylpyrrolidone.

3.2 Properties of crospovidone

3.2.1 Description, specifications, pharmacopoeias

3.2.1.1 *Description*

The crospovidone grades of Table 113 are products of pharmaceutical quality obtained according to the cGMP regulations. They are white or almost white powders with a porous structure and a large surface area. The normal grades, and, to a lesser extent, the micronized or fine powder grades have good flow properties. Since the products are insoluble, they can be thoroughly washed with water to achieve a very high degree of purity.

The products have practically no taste or odour.

One of the main properties of crospovidone is its complete insolubility in all the usual solvents.

3.2.1.2
Pharmacopoeial requirements

The products are tested and released in accordance with the methods and limits given in the monographs "Crospovidone" of USP26-NF21 and of Ph.Eur. (Normal grades of Table 113 = Type A, micronized powders of Table 113 = Type B). Crospovidone also meet the requirements of the monograph "Crospovidone" of the Japanese Pharmaceutical Excipients (JPE) (Table 115).

All crospovidone grades meet the ICH requirements on residual solvents according to Ph.Eur., 5.4: No residual solvents (class 1–3) are likely to be present. Furthermore they meat the requirements for organic volatile impurities of USP 26.

The microbial status can be determined according to Ph.Eur. methods 2.6.12 and 2.6.13. The limits given in the European Pharmacopoeia (Table 116) apply.

Table 115. Current pharmacopoeial requirements for crospovidone

	Normal crospovidone	Micronized crospovidone
Identity (see also 3.3.1.1)	Passes test (Type A)	Passes test (Type B)
Nitrogen (%, see 2.3.3.7)	12.0–12.8	12.0–12.8
Water (K. Fischer, %) USP-NF	≤ 5.0	≤ 5.0
Loss on drying (%) Ph. Eur.	≤ 5.0	≤ 5.0
pH (1% in water)	5.0–7.5	5.0–7.5
Vinylpyrrolidone (HPLC*, ppm)	≤ 10	≤ 10
Sulfated ash (%)	≤ 0.1	≤ 0.1
Heavy metals (ppm)	≤ 10	≤ 10
Soluble components (%)	≤ 1.0	≤ 1.0
Peroxides (ppm H_2O_2)	≤ 400	≤ 1000
Residual solvents	Not present	Not present
Microbial status (see Table 116)	Passes test	Passes test

* Methods see Sections 3.3.2.2 and 3.3.2.3

Table 116. Microbial purity requirements (Ph.Eur. 5, 5.1.4, Category 2 + 3A)

- Max. 10^2 aerobic bacteria and fungi/g
- No Escherichia coli/g
- Max. 10^1 enterobacteria and other gramnegative bacteria/g
- No Pseudomonas aeruginosa/g
- No Staphylococcus aureus/g

3.2.2
Particle size, bulk density

3.2.2.1
Particle size distribution

The particle size distribution and its effect on the flow and swelling properties of crospovidone are an important factor in its use in solid pharmaceutical preparations. A relatively fine particle size minimizes the changes in the tablet surface as a result of atmospheric humidity and swelling, although large particles, with their greater swelling volume, would have given more rapid disintegration.

The crospovidone monograph of Ph.Eur. 5 requires a functional classification into Type A (= non-micronized product) and Type B (= micronized product) by means of a particle size measurement in identification test D.

The best method of the determination of the particle size distribution of the different crospovidone types is the light diffraction measurement (e.g. Malvern Master Sizer, see Fig. 63 and 64). The particle size distribution of normal crospovidone also can be measured by sieving or air jet screening. In this dry sieving method more than 50 % of the particles are coarser than 50 µm without any swelling. Therefore even with this dry method it corresponds clearly to the definition of Type A of the Ph.Eur. monograph.

The particle size distribution of micronized crospovidone can be measured as suspension in water or cyclohexane by a Malvern Master Sizer and there is no significant influence of the solvent. If almost all particles are finer than 50 µm it is classified as Type B of Ph.Eur.

Figure 64 shows typical results for the micronized powder grades of the market.

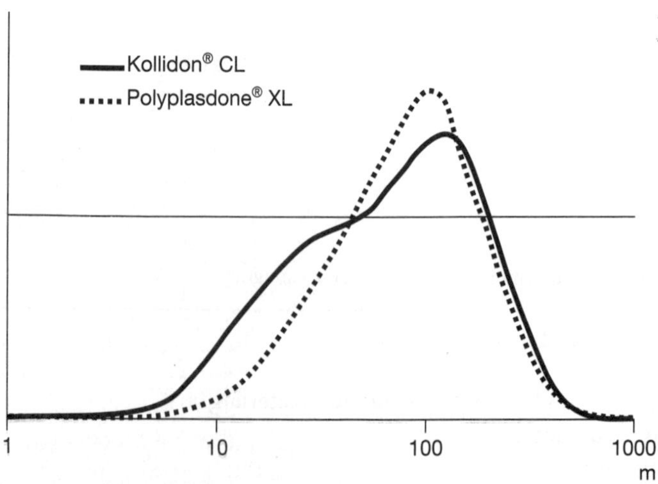

Fig. 63. Particle size distribution of the normal grades of crospovidone available in the market (Method: Malvern Master Sizer)

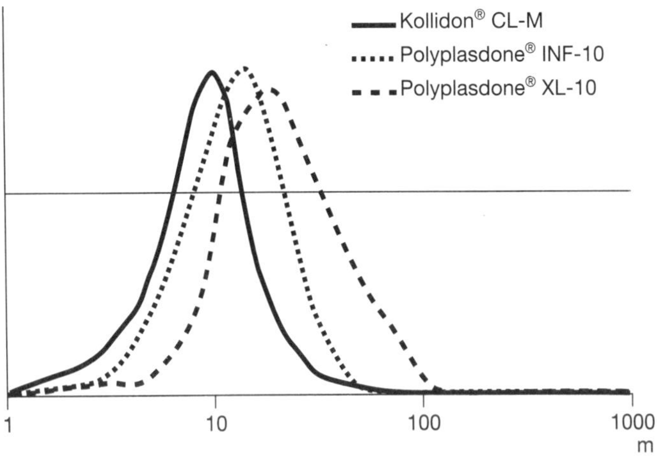

Fig. 64. Particle size distribution of the micronized/fine powder grades of crospovidone available in the market (Method: Malvern Master Sizer)

3.2.2.2
Particle structure

Crospovidone has the typical morphology of a popcorn polymer. The Figs. 65 and 66 illustrate the particle structure of the normal and the micronized products in form of scanning electron photomicrographs. These graphs also show the strong difference of particle size between these two types of crospovidone because both figures have an identical magnification.

3.2.2.3
Bulk density, tap density

Table 117 gives the typical values for the bulk density and tap density for all crospovidone grades available in the market. The major differences in the bulk densities of the micronized/fine powder grades have an important effect on their applications.

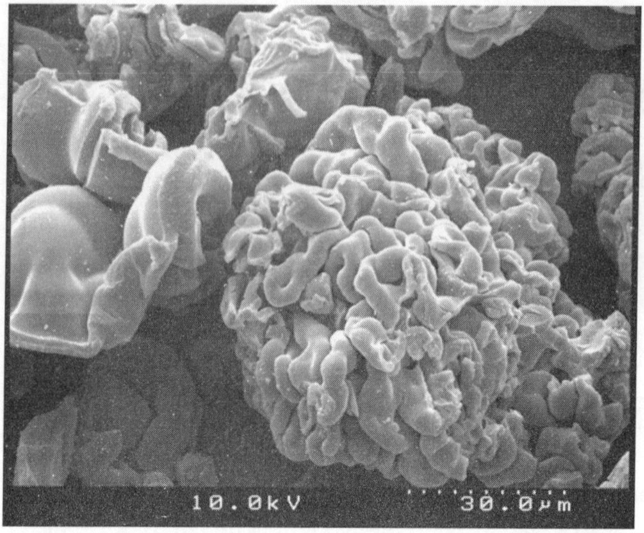

Fig. 65. Typical pop-corn structure of normal crospovidone (Ph.Eur. Type A)

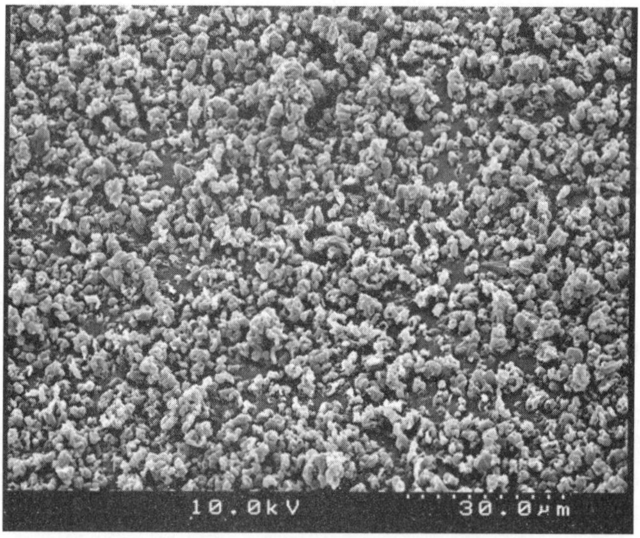

Fig. 66. Typical particle structure of micronized crospovidone (Ph.Eur. Type B)

Table 117. Typical bulk densities and tap densities of the crospovidone grades available in the market

Trade name	Bulk density	Tap density
Normal grades:		
Kollidon® CL	about 0.35 g/ml	about 0.45 g/ml
Polyplasdone® XL	about 0.2 g/ml	about 0.3 g/ml
Micronized/fine powder grades:		
Kollidon®CL-M	about 0.2 g/ml	about 0.3 g/ml
Polyplasdone® XL-10	about 0.3 g/ml	about 0.5 g/ml
Polyplasdone® INF-10	about 0.4 g/ml	about 0.5 g/ml

3.2.3 Specific surface area, water absorption

3.2.3.1 *Specific surface area*

The crospovidone grades are obtained with different specific surface areas, depending on the polymerization conditions, and their particle size. The micronization process has less influence on the specific surface than small modifications of the polymerization conditions. When a normal crospovidone was micronized the specific surface only increased from 1 m^2/g to 1.8 m^2/g (N_2-BET method). The micronized crospovidone of the lowest bulk density available in the market has the highest specific surface of 2.5 to 6 m^2/g (Table 118).

Table 118. Specific surface area of crospovidone available in the market [662]

Crospovidone grade	Specific surface area
Normal grades:	
Kollidon® CL	0.95 m^2/g
Polyplasdone® XL	0.85 m^2/g
Micronized grades:	
Kollidon® CL-M	2.37 m^2/g
Polyplasdone® XL-10	1.00 m^2/g

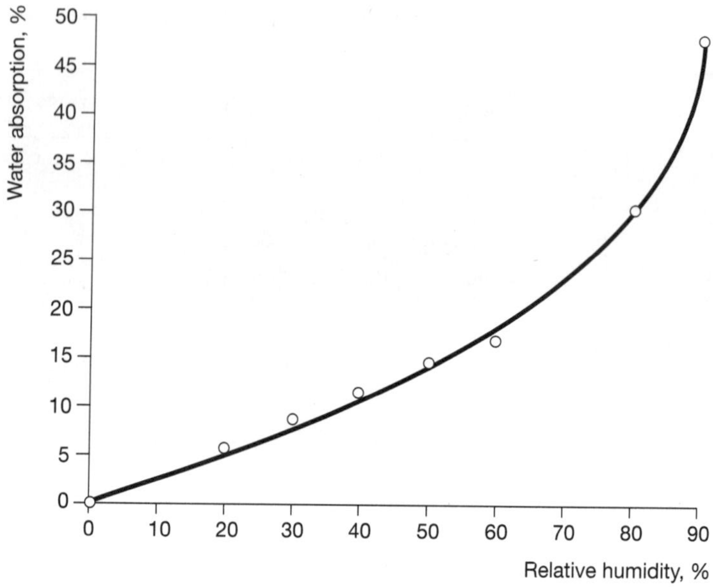

Fig. 67. Water absorption by crospovidone at 25°C after 7 days

3.2.3.2
Hygroscopicity

Crospovidone is almost as hygroscopic as povidone. It has not been possible to find any significant difference in water adsorption between the different grades of crospovidone, so that Fig. 67 applies for all grades.

3.2.3.3
Hydration

If water is added to crospovidone instead of merely exposing it to atmospheric humidity, it binds significantly more. Its hydration capacity is best determined by the following method [3]:

> Add 2.0 g of crospovidone to 40 ml of water in a 100-ml centrifuge tube and shake vigorously until a suspension is obtained. Shake up again after 5 and after 10 minutes. Then centrifuge for 15 minutes at 2000 rpm. Decant off the supernatant liquid. Then reweigh.

The hydration capacity is calculated as the quotient of the weight after hydration and the initial weight. For normal crospovidone, usually it lies in the range 3–6.

3.2.4 Swelling

One of the most important properties of crospovidone in its applications is its ability to swell in a predictable manner without forming a gel. A number of methods are described in the literature for measuring swelling, the most important being listed in Table 119.

The swelling pressure of crospovidone varies from grade to grade. Fig. 68 shows the swelling pressures of one of the normal and one of the micronized crospovidone types (lightly compacted 1.5 kN) in three different solvents for comparison. Practically no difference emerged between ethanol and water.

Table 119. Some methods for determining the swelling of crospovidone

- Swelling pressure of lightly compacted powder (see Fig. 68)
- Swelling volume of compacted powder [392]
- Swelling volume of the particles in the Coulter Counter [221]
- Swelling volume of the particles under the microscope
- Water adsorption with and without magnesium stearate [392, 394]
- Water binding capacity [3]
- Water adsorption in placebo tablets [262]
- Swelling volume in placebo tablets [392]
- Swelling pressure of placebo tablets [395]
- Disintegration force with placebo tablets [391, 398, 399]

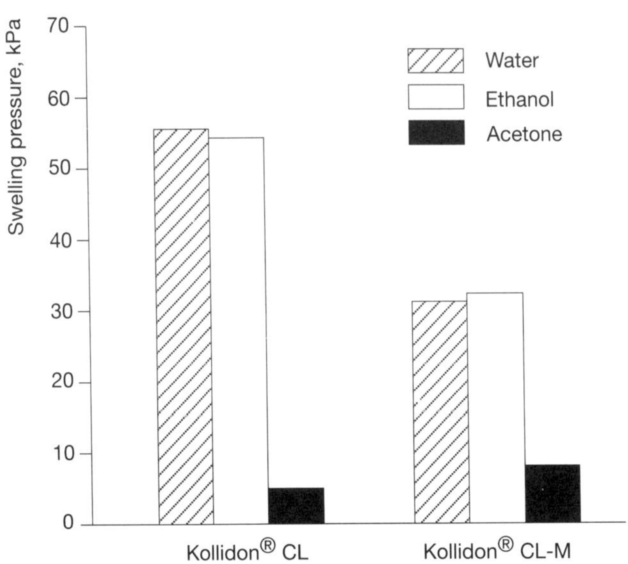

Fig. 68. Swelling pressure of two lightly compacted types of crospovidone in different solvents

The swelling pressure of the normal crospovidone type in water is about twice as high as that of the micronized product.

In nonpolar solvents such as cyclohexane, hexane, dioxane and ethyl acetate, crospovidone hardly swells at all. Even in acetone it swells much less than in water, as can be seen from Fig. 68. In 0.1 N hydrochloric acid too, it swells significantly less than in isotonic salt solution [221].

3.2.5 Complexation, chemical interactions

3.2.5.1 *Complexation*

As with povidone, crospovidone also forms chemical complexes or associates with a large number of drugs and other substances. For a typical example of comparison see Section 3.4.3.1. Here, too, the formation of the complexes is reversible and they do not form in alkaline medium. Whether crospovidone forms a complex with a drug depends on its chemical structure.

Systematic investigations of aromatic compounds have shown that phenol and carboxyl groups have a strong influence on complexation. This is shown in Fig. 69.

For most drugs, the degree of complexation lies within the range that provides an acceleration in dissolution rate.

Normally, the degree of complexation is so low that, at best, an acceleration in the dissolution of the drug can be observed (see Section 3.4.3). The complexation constants of a number of active substances in 0.1 N hydrochloric acid can be seen in Table 120. They were also determined by adsorption on crospovidone in 0.01 N hydrochloric acid and, in some cases, in synthetic gastric juice according to USP [158].

The complexation constants can be used in Fig. 70 to estimate any adverse effects of the adsorption of a drug on its release and absorption by the body. Figure 70 covers the range of drug concentrations encountered in practice.

The shaded area in Fig. 70 shows the usual systemic concentration range of crospovidone after medication. Thus for a complexation constant of less than 20 l mol-1, the bound portion of the drug is always considerably less than 10%. Tannin and hexylresorcinol are exceptions with higher complexation constants [158]. Catechin also has a complexation constant of more than 1000 l mol-1. Certain halogen compounds may have complexation constants in excess of 20 l mol^{-1}.

That complexes are formed only in the acidic range is shown for resorcinol in Fig. 71.

As with povidone, the ability of crospovidone to form complexes, as an auxiliary or as an active substance in its own right, is widely used in pharmaceuticals (Table 121).

The complex formation capacity of individual batches of crospovidone can be measured in terms of their adsorption of salicylic acid (see Section 3.3.3).

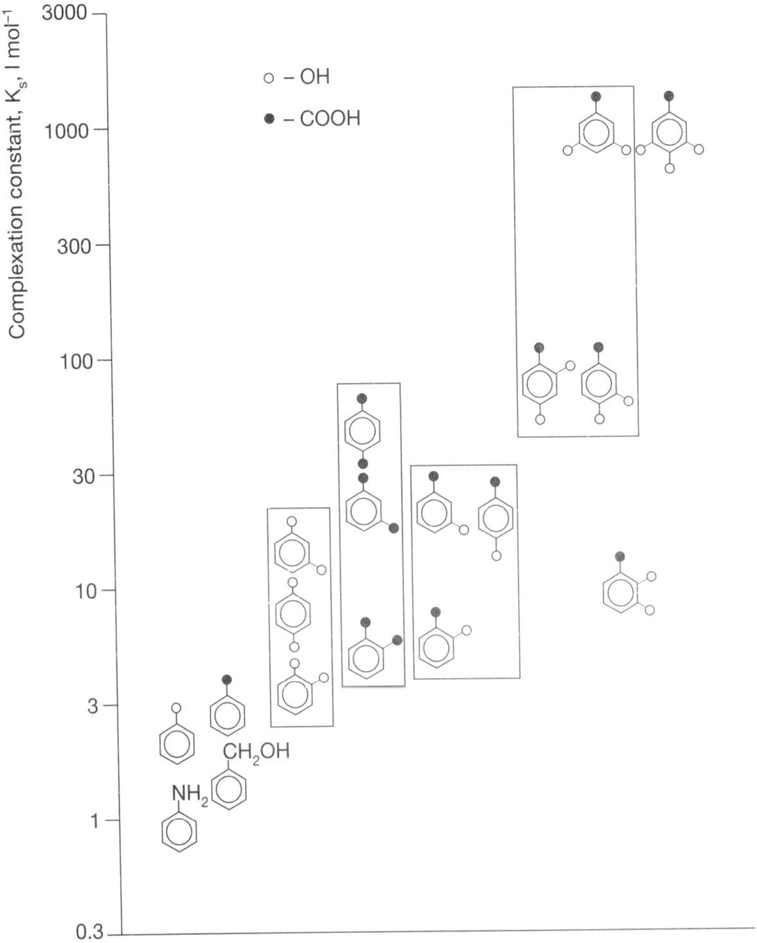

Fig. 69. Influence of the structure of aromatic compounds on their formation of complexes with crospovidone [192]

Table 120. Complexation constants for some drugs and other substances with crospovidone in 0.1 N hydrochloric acid [192]

Substance	Complexation constant, K_S, l mol^{-1}
Acetaminophen (paracetamol)	2.0
Acetylsalicylic acid	1.5
Benzocaine	1.9
Benzoic acid	2.9
Chloramphenicol	≈ 0
Caffeine	≈ 0
alpha-Methyldopa	0.2

▶

Table 120. Continued

Substance	Complexation constant, K_s, l mol^{-1}
Methylparaben	4.2
Papaverine HCl	0.1
Promethazine HCl	0.4
Resorcinol	13.1
Riboflavin	≈ 0
Salicylamide	3.7
Salicylic acid	6.2
Sorbic acid	0.5
Sulfamethazine	≈ 0
Sulfamoxole	≈ 0
Sulfathiazole	1.0
Tannin	>1000
Tetracaine HCl	≈ 0
Trimethoprim	≈ 0

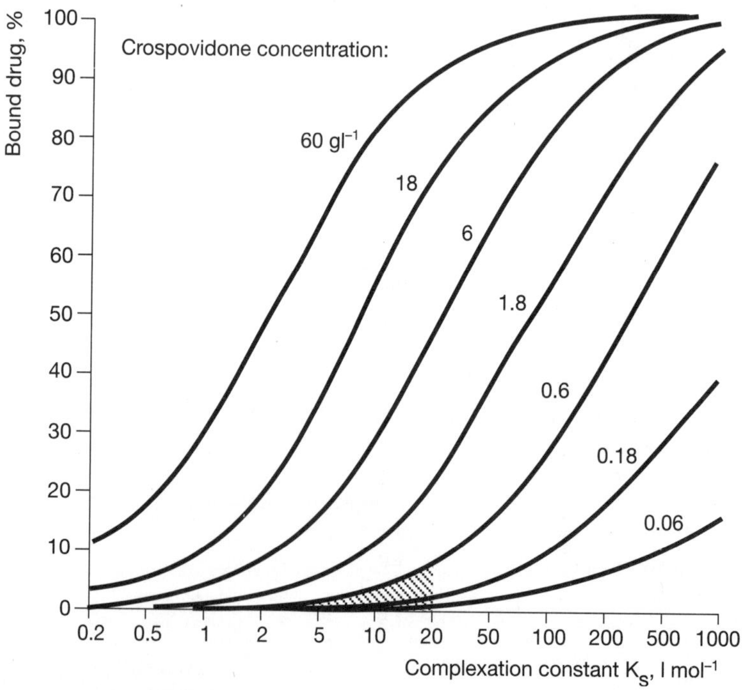

Fig. 70. Family of curves for the proportion of bound drug as a function of the complexation constant, K_s at different crospovidone concentrations [192]

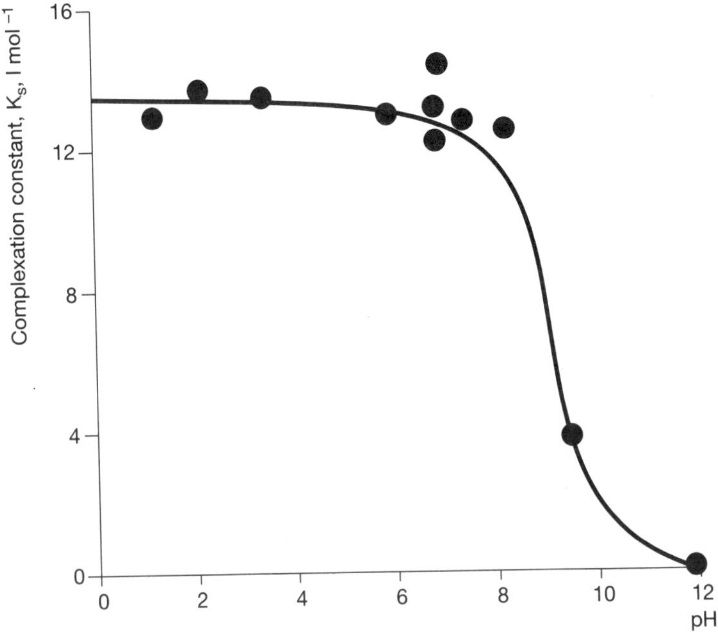

Fig. 71. Effect of pH value on the complex between resorcinol and crospovidone [192]

Table 121. Applications of normal and micronized crospovidone as complexing agent in drugs

1. Improvement of the dissolution and bioavailability of drugs (Sections 3.4.2 and 3.4.3)
2. Active substance against diarrhoea, gastritis, ulcers and hiatus hernia (Section 3.4.5)
3. Adsorption and removal of the polyphenols and tannins from tinctures and plant extracts (Section 3.4.6)
4. Improvement of the taste of acetaminophen (see Table 143), of azithromycin and some other drug substances

3.2.5.2
Chemical interactions

Crospovidone can contain small quantities of peroxides, within the limits of the specifications, which could theoretically react with drugs in exceptional cases. However, no evidence of this has been found in practice. On the contrary, it has been observed that the vitamins in multivitamin drink granulates were stabilized by micronized crospovidone (see Section 3.4.6.2).

3.2.6
Stability, storage, packaging

3.2.6.1
Stability of the pure products

Crospovidone has a shelf life of more than three years, after which the different types still meet the specifications given in Table 115, when they are stored in the original, sealed containers at room temperature (20–25 °C).

3.2.6.2
Stability in finished pharmaceuticals

Crospovidone also demonstrates excellent stability after processing into tablets, granules, capsules or suspensions, so that no changes are to be expected over many years. However, it should be borne in mind that the products are hygroscopic, so that if there are any leaks in the packaging, through which atmospheric humidity can enter, the crospovidone particles may swell. Tablets made from such product have a rough surface.

The peroxide formation in placebo tablets (400 mg microcrystalline cellulose, 20 mg crospovidone, 3 mg magnesium stearate) was studied at room temperature over a storage period of 2 years. The results given in Table 122 show that no significant amounts of peroxides was formed in the tablets during this storage period.

Table 122. Peroxide formation in placebo tablets containing 5 % of crospovidone during storage at 20–25°C

Storage time	Peroxide level
Initial value	1 ppm
6 Months	8 ppm
12 Months	3 ppm
18 Months	4 ppm
24 Months	3 ppm

3.3 Analytical methods for crospovidone

3.3.1 Qualitative and quantitative methods of determination

3.3.1.1 *Identification*

The Pharmacopoeias and the literature describe only three detection reactions for the identification of crospovidone.

The most important and clearest method of identification is by infrared spectroscopy. The same method can be used for all the types of crospovidone. Figure 72 shows this infrared spectrum. The only disadvantage of this method of identification is that soluble polyvinylpyrrolidone (povidone) gives the same infrared spectrum (see Section 2.3.1.1, Fig. 24). However, the difference can readily be determined from the solubility.

In an alternative method, 0.1 ml of 0.1 N iodine solution is added to a suspension of 1 g of crospovidone in 10 ml of water. After vigorous shaking, 1 ml of starch solution is added. The iodine is complexed by the crospovidone, so that no blue coloration develops within 30 seconds.

The fact that crospovidone do not dissolve in any solvent provides a further indication of identity.

The crospovidone monograph of Ph.Eur. requires as identification D a functional classification of crospovidone into Type A (= non-micronized product) and Type B (= micronized product) by means of a particle size measurement.

This classification was developed by the laboratory of Ph.Eur. measuring samples of different crospovidones as agueous suspensions in water and observing the swollen particles under the microscope. It was found that in the case of the tested micronized product almost 100% of the particles were finer than 50 µm (= definition of Type B) and that in the case of the non-micronized product more than 50% (= the majority) were coarser than 50 µm (= definiton of Type A) [631].

3.3.1.2 *Quantitative determination of crospovidone*

Crospovidone can be quantitatively determined by two methods.

1. *Nitrogen determination*

The nitrogen content is determined by the method of the monograph "Crospovidone" of USP26-NF21 or Ph.Eur. 5 (for the detailed method see also Section 2.3.3.7). The theoretical value is 12.6%.

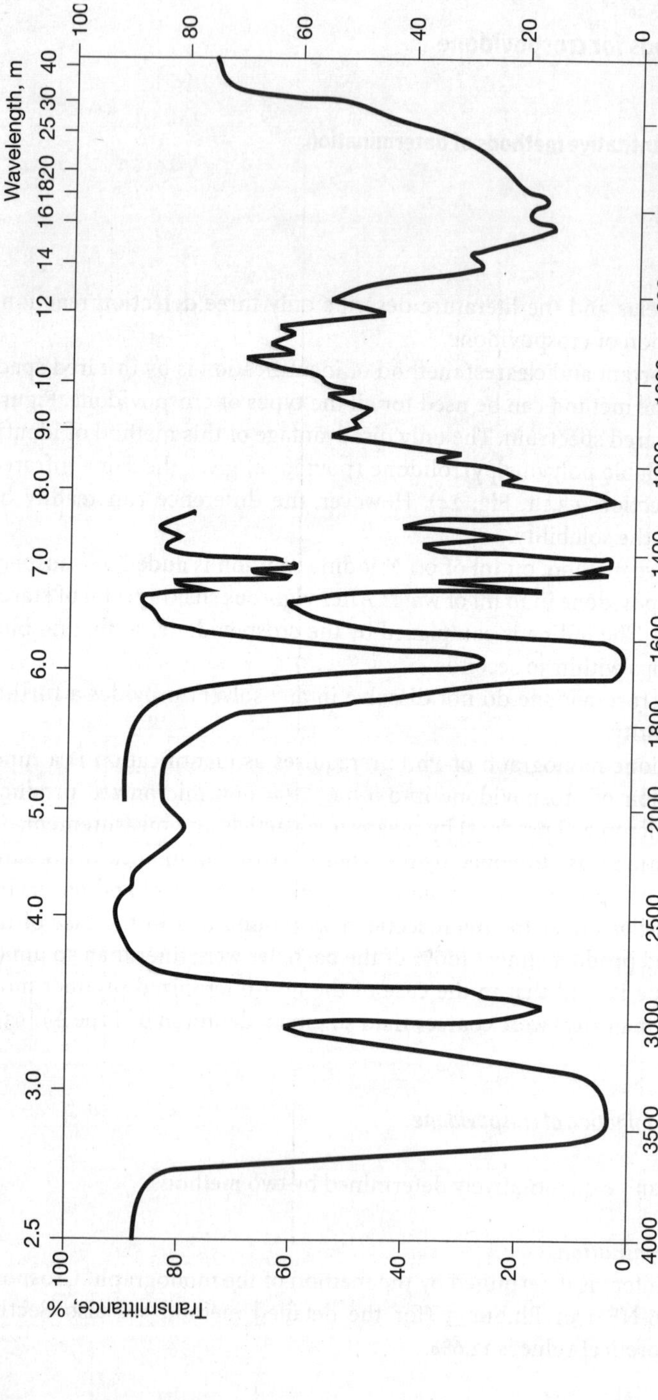

Fig. 72. Infrared spectrum of crospovidone recorded in potassium bromide

Table 123. Purity test methods for crospovidone decribed in the Pharmacopoeias (2004)

Classification as Type A or Type B by the particle size (only Ph. Eur.)
Monomer (N-vinylpyrrolidone = impurity A)
Water-soluble compounds
Peroxides (different limits for Type A and Type B)
Water/loss on drying
Sulphated ash
Heavy metals
Nitrogen
Residual solvents/Organic volatible impurities

2. *Gravimetric determination*
Accurately weigh a sample of crospovidone, thoroughly wash with water and dry for 3 hours at 105 °C. The final weight must be more than 98% of the initial weight, calculated for the dried substance.

3.3.2 Methods for the determination of purity

3.3.2.1 *Pharmacopoeia methods*

The methods for the determination of the purity of crospovidone are described in detail in the United States Pharmacopoeia (USP 26-NF 21) and the European Pharmacopoeia (Ph.Eur. 5). They cover all the parameters listed in Table 123.

The tests for hydrazine and 2-pyrrolidone, which are specified by the Pharmacopoeias for povidone, are not required for crospovidone, as these impurities are not present. Also residual solvents or organic volatile impurities are not present.

3.3.2.2 *HPLC method for the determination of free N-vinylpyrrolidone*

As crospovidone grades contains levels of N-vinylpyrrolidone that lie well below the detection limit of the iodometric titration method given in the crospovidone monograph of USP26-NF21, it is recommended to employ a more sentitive method such as high performance liquid chromatography as now included in the crospovidone monograph of Ph.Eur. or gas chromatography (see section 3.3.2.3). These chromatographic methods have proved both accurate and precise.

An HPLC method with a detection limit of less than 1 ppm of N-vinylpyrrolidone is given below. It is the method mentioned in the crospovidone monograph of Ph.Eur. 5.

Principle
An extract of the sample is separated by reversed phase chromatography. The interfering polymeric matrix is removed by switching columns. A UV detector operating at 235 nm, calibrated with an external standard, is used to determine the level of monomer.

Sample preparation
Weigh about 800 mg of crospovidone, accurate to 0.1 mg, into a conical flask, add 25 ml of the mobile phase and shake for 60 minutes. After the particles have settled filtrate through a 0.2 μm filter. Aliquots of this solution are used for the HPLC analysis.

If the N-vinylpyrrolidone content would exceed 10 ppm, the sample weight should be reduced or the solution diluted accordingly.

Preparation of the calibration solution
Weigh 40–50 mg of N-vinylpyrrolidone, accurate to 0.01 mg, into a 50-ml volumetric flask and dissolve in about 20 ml of eluent. Then make up to the mark with eluent.

Prepare a dilution series from this stock solution to cover the range in which the N-vinylpyrrolidone content of the crospovidone sample is expected (Table 124).

Column switching
The analysis is started with the guard column and separation column in series. After about 3 min, the valves, controlled by the detector programme, switch over such that the eluent flows past the guard column, direct to the separation column. The columns are switched at a point when the components to be determined, but not the interfering matrix, have reached the separation column. After about 35

Table 124. Chromatographic conditions

Guard column:	25 x 4 mm cartridge packed with LiChrospher® 60 RP select B, 5 μm (Merck)
Separation column:	250 x 4 mm steel column packed with LiChrospher 60 RP select B, 5 μm (Merck)
Eluent (mobile phase):	Water/acetonitrile (92 + 8% wt.)
Flow rate:	1 ml/min
Sample volume:	20 μl
Detection wavelength:	235 nm
Column temperature:	Room temperature
Retention time:	Approx. 11 min

min the columns are washed out in the reverse direction by a second pump, to remove the unwanted matrix components (0–10 min: eluent + acetonitrile 3 + 7; after 10 min: only acetonitrile).

If a detector without a programming option is used, switching can be carried out manually or by another programmable component, e.g. the pump.

Calculation

1. *Calibration factor:*

$$F = \frac{A_C}{W_{St}}$$

A_C = calibration substance peak area [mV s]
W_{St} = weight of calibration substance per 100 ml [mg/100 ml]

2. *N-Vinylpyrrolidone in the sample*

The content of the sample is calculated with the aid of an external standard:

$$\text{ppm N-vinylpyrrolidone} = \frac{A}{F\,W_{Sa}}\ 10^6$$

A = peak area [mV s]
W_{Sa} = sample weight [mg/100 ml]

Validation

Linearity

The calibration curve was plotted from 7 points covering a concentration range of 0.01 to 11.0 μg/ml to check the linearity. Figure 73 shows the calibration curve obtained.

Reproducibility

The N-vinylpyrrolidone content of a sample was determined six times. The values found and the average are given in Table 125.

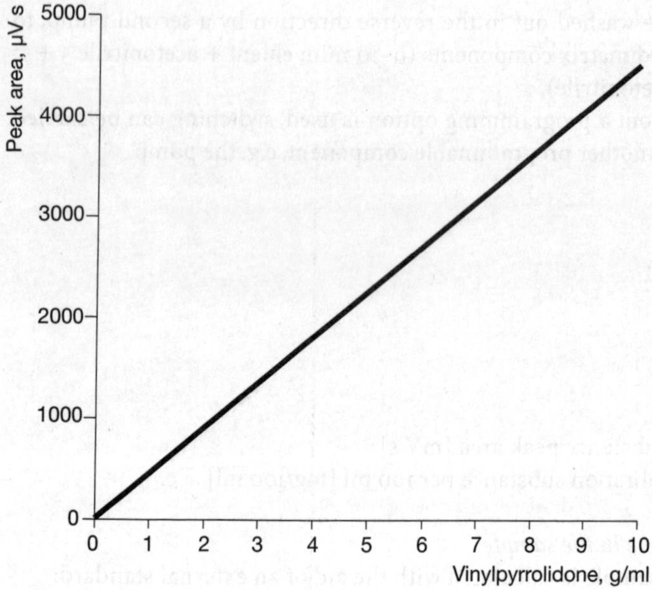

Fig. 73. Calibration curve for the HPLC determination of N-vinylpyrrolidone

Table 125. N-Vinylpyrrolidone content of a sample (1992)

Determination No.	N-vinylpyrrolidone [mg/kg]
1	15.0
2	15.5
3	15.0
4	15.4
5	15.4
6	15.4
Average	15.3

3.3.2.3
Gas chromatography determination of free N-vinylpyrrolidone in crospovidone

As an alternative to HPLC, it is also possible to use gas chromatography to determine free vinylpyrrolidone. The following method has a detection limit of 2 ppm.

Principle
The acetone extract of the polymer is analyzed by gas chromatography, using N-(3-methoxypropyl)pyrrolidone as an internal standard. A nitrogen-specific detector (NSD) is used.

Table 126. Gas chromatographic conditions

Temperatures:	
– Column oven	170 °C
– Injection block	220 °C
– Detector	220 °C
Carrier gas:	Helium, 38 ml/min
Detector conditions (nitrogen-specific detector):	
– Air	300 ml/min
– Hydrogen	30 ml/min
Sample volume: 1 μl of the supernatant solution	

Standard solution
Dissolve 200 mg of N-(3-methoxypropyl)pyrrolidone, weighed accurate to 0.2 mg, in 100 ml of acetone.

Apparatus
Gas chromatograph with NSD and 1.0-m glass column of inside diameter approx. 2.0 mm, packed with 5% KOH and 15% Polypropylene Glycol 2025 (available from Merck-Schuchardt) on kieselguhr (45/60 mesh, Perkin-Elmer).

Gas chromatography analysis
Sample preparation: weigh 2.0–2.5 g, accurate to 0.2 mg, of crospovidone into a 50-ml flask. Add 1 ml of standard solution with a one-mark pipette. Then mix with approx. 25 ml of acetone, shake for 4 hours and, when the polymer has settled out, analyze the supernatant solution by gas chromatography (Table 126).

Factor determination
Weigh about 200 mg of vinylpyrrolidone and 2 g of N-(methoxypropyl)-pyrrolidone, accurate to 0.2 mg, into a 100-ml volumetric flask and dissolve in acetone to make 100 ml. Transfer 1.0 ml of the solution to a further 100-ml volumetric flask with a pipette and dilute to 100 ml with acetone (= calibration solution).

Calibrate the apparatus by analyzing three 1.0-µl samples of independently prepared calibration solutions.

$$F = \frac{W\ A_{MPP}}{W_{MPP}\ A}$$

where,

W = weight of vinylpyrrolidone [mg]
W_{MPP} = weight of N-(3-methoxypropyl)pyrrolidone [mg]
A = peak area for vinylpyrrolidone (area units or mV· s)

A_{MPP} = peak area for N-(3-methoxypropyl)pyrrolidone (peak area units or mV·s)
The factor, F should be checked daily.

Calculation of the content (Fig. 74)

$$\text{ppm N-vinylpyrrolidone} = \frac{1000\ F\ C_{St}\ A}{W_S\ A_{MPP}}$$

where,
F = factor
C_{St} = N-(methoxypropyl)pyrrolidone concentration of the standard solution [mg/ml]
A = peak area for vinylpyrrolidone (area units or mV s)
W_S = sample weight [g]
A_{MPP} = peak area for N-(3-methoxypropyl)pyrrolidone (area units or mV s)

Validation against the HPLC method (Ph.Eur. 5)

For the release of crospovidone sometimes this GC method is preferred instead of the HPLC method prescribed in the "Crospovidone" monograph of Ph.Eur. because the components vinylpyrrolidone and 2-pyrrolidone can be determined in one GC chromatogram and the use of methanol can be avoided.

The following results show the equivalence of the results obtained by both methods.

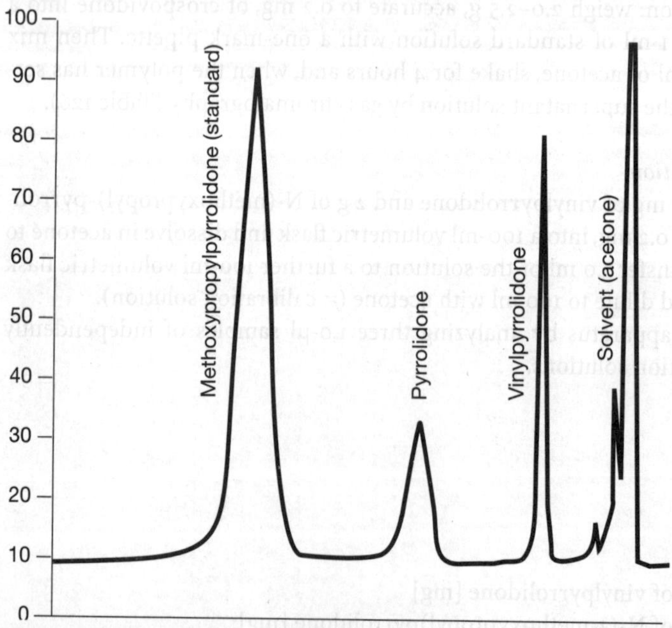

Fig. 74. Gas chromatogram for vinylpyrrolidone, pyrrolidone and the internal standard

Reproducibility of both methods
The trials shown in Table 127 were done with batch 1696/10 of the crospovidone type Kollidon® CL.

Recovery rate of the GC method
The trials shown in Table 128 were done with the same batch 1696/10 used in the trials of reproducibility (Table 127).

Comparison of both methods on different batches
The trials shown in Table 129 were done with different batches. They illustrate that both methods give comparable results.

Table 127. Comparison of GC and HPLC on one batch of crospovidone

Sample	GC Date	GC Result (mg/kg)	HPLC (Ph. Eur.) Date	HPLC (Ph. Eur.) Result (mg/kg)
1	28.3.02	5,2	15.4.02	5,1
2	28.3.02	5,5	15.4.02	5,1
3	15.4.02	5,6	15.4.02	5,1
4	15.4.02	5,7	15.4.02	5,2
5	15.4.02	5,6	15.4.02	5,1

Table 128. Recovery of the gas chromatographic method on crospovidone

Trial	Initial value mg/kg	Added amount mg/kg	Theoretical mg/kg	Found mg/kg	Recovery rate %
1	5,5	1,0	6,5	6,8	130,0
2	5,5	3,0	8,5	8,7	106,7
3	5,5	5,0	10,5	11,3	116,0
4	5,5	6,1	11,6	11,8	103,3
5	5,5	9,9	15,4	16,2	108,1

Table 129. Comparison of GC and HPLC on five batches of crospovidone

Batch	GC Date	GC Result (mg/kg)	HPLC (Ph. Eur.) Date	HPLC (Ph. Eur.) Result (mg/kg)
1688/10	16.4.02	3,4	4.4.02	3,1
1693/10	25.3.02	1,8	15.4.02	1,4
1694/10	25.3.02	8,1	15.4.02	7,4
1696/10	28.3.02	5,2	15.4.02	5,1
1697/10	28.3.02	10,1	15.4.02	9,5

3.3.3
Determination of the complexation capacity with salicylic acid

Salicylic acid has been selected as a model substance to provide a standard method for measuring the complexation capacity of crospovidone. Measurement of the complex formation constant for this substance in water gave a value of 4.1 l . mol^{-1} [158].

The following method measures the percentage of salicylic acid that is complexed by a given quantity of crospovidone. The value normally lies between 30% and 50% at 20 °C.

Preparation of the 0.1 N salicylic acid solution
Dissolve 13.81 g of salicylic acid in 500 ml of methanol in a 1000-ml volumetric flask and make up almost to the mark with water. After 24 hours at 23–25°C, make up exactly to the mark.

Procedure
Accurately weigh about 2 g of crospovidone into a conical flask (sample weight = W).

Calculate the volume of 0.1 N salicylic acid solution required, taking into account the water content, w of the product to be tested, with the following formula:

$$\text{Volume (ml)} = \frac{W\ (g) \times 43 \times (100 - w\ [\%]}{100} \quad (= \text{approx. } 80)$$

Transfer the calculated volume of 0.1 N salicylic acid solution to the conical flask, close and shake vigorously for 5 min at 23–25°C. Fill the resulting suspension non-quantitatively into centrifuge tubes, and centrifuge for 10 min at 4000 rpm.

Filter the supernatant solution through a No. 4 glass frit covered by a paper filter. Titrate exactly 20 ml of the clear or opalescent filtrate against 0.1 N sodium hydroxide solution, using phenolphthalein as indicator (titre in ml = t).

To obtain the 100-% value, titrate exactly 20 ml of 0.1 N salicylic acid solution against 0.1 N sodium hydroxide solution in the same manner (titre in ml = T).

Calculation
Calculate the complexed salicylic acid with the following formula:

$$\% \text{ complexed} = \frac{(T - t)\ 100}{T}$$

3.3.4 Quantitative determination of crospovidone in preparations

Gravimetric analysis provides the best method for the quantitative determination of normal crospovidone in preparations.

Principle
Suspend the sample material in water and/or a suitable solvent that dissolves all the other components of the preparation. Crospovidone is determined gravimetrically after filtration and drying.

Procedure
Accurately weigh about 5 g of sample, that contains 2–5% of crospovidone, into a glass beaker and mix with about 250 ml of water or other solvent. Insert a magnetic stirrer bar and cover the beaker with a clock glass. Stir for 2 hours.

Then leave to settle and draw off the supernatant solution through a dried and preweighed G 4 Gooch crucible. Wash and leave to stand again, decant the supernatant solution through the Gooch crucible, then quantitatively transfer the residue to the Gooch crucible with small portions of water.

Dry at 105 °C for 3 hours.

Calculation
The content is given as a percentage by the following formula:

$$\%\ \text{Crospovidone} = \frac{\text{Weight after filtration [g]} \times 100}{\text{Original sample weight [g]}}$$

3.4 Applications of crospovidone

3.4.1 General application properties

Crospovidone possess a series of properties that are used in the manufacture of different pharmaceutical products and dosage forms (Table 130).

The most important property of crospovidone as an auxiliary is its *disintegration and dissolution enhancing effect*, which can be used in tablets, granules and hard gelatin capsules

Its ability to form *complexes* is useful in solid and liquid dosage forms.

The improvement brought about by crospovidone in the dissolution of insoluble drugs is particularly useful for tablets and granules.

The use of micronized/fine powder crospovidone as an active substance against diarrhoea depends on its ability to form complexes, as does the use of crospovidone ("PVPP") in removing polyphenols from wine, beer and plant extracts. The

Table 130. Functions and properties of crospovidone as excipient

- Acceleration of tablet disintegration and therefore also of dissolution and bioavailability of the active substances as a result of predictable swelling (disintegration effect)
- Improvement of dissolution and bioavailability of insoluble drugs by complex formation
- Selective adsorption of polyphenols by complex formation
- Stabilization of suspensions by low-density micronized crospovidone as a hydrophilic polymer
- Stabilization of vitamins
- Adsorption of endotoxins by complexation
- Adsorption of water (desiccant)
- Taste masking of acetaminophen, azithromycin etc.

ability of micronized crospovidone of low density to *stabilize suspensions* finds its most important application in antibiotics, antacids and vitamin preparations.

The hygroscopicity of crospovidone (see Section 3.2.3.2) can be used to *adsorb water* in preparations that contain moisture-sensitive drugs, to improve their stability. It almost certainly also contributes to the efficacy of micronized/fine powder crospovidone as an active substance in the treatment of diarrhoea.

3.4.2 Crospovidone as disintegrant and dissolution agent for tablets, granules and hard gelatin capsules

3.4.2.1 *General*

The active ingredient of a tablet must be bioavailable. To achieve or improve this, one must be aware of the following sequence of events after the tablet is taken (Table 131).

The disintegration of the tablet or the capsule can be regarded as the first step on the path to bioavailability and to the pharmacological action of the drug taking effect. To achieve this, it is usually necessary to add a disintegrant to the tablet.

Different disintegrants work in different ways, which can involve swelling, wicking and deformation effects, and the repulsion of charged particles. The effect of crospovidone as a disintegrant is based mainly on its predictable swelling properties (see Section 3.2.4).

Table 131. How the drug in a tablet becomes bioavailable

Ingestion

↓

Disintegration of the tablet or capsule in the gastric or intestinal juice

↓

Distribution of the particles in the gastrointestinal tract

↓

Dissolution of the drug in the gastric or intestinal juice

↓

Absorption of the drug by the mucous membrane of the stomach or intestine

3.4.2.2
Quantities and processing

The optimum quantity of crospovidone in a tablet or in granules is specific to each particular formulation and cannot be predicted accurately. It also depends very much on the desired disintegration time, which is different for an analgesic than for a coated multivitamin tablet. In practice it has been found that the usual concentration lies in the 1–5% range. If the proportion is increased beyond 5%, the disintegration time is frequently no longer improved by a worthwhile amount. With the placebo tablets consisting of calcium hydrogen phosphate and lactose (3 + 1), which were used to measure the values in Fig. 75, as little as 1% of disintegrant was sufficient to reduce the disintegration time to less than 5 minutes.

In difficult cases, such as griseofulvin tablets, however, a higher proportion of crospovidone can provide a significant improvement [93].

Apart from the proportion of the disintegrant, the method by which it is incorporated and the point at which it is added to the tabletting mixture also play a certain role.

Methods Nos. 1 and 2 in Table 132, in which the disintegrant is added after granulation, are used most frequently. In Methods Nos. 3 and 4, the disintegrant is added prior to granulation, while in Nos. 5 and 6 part of the disintegrant is added before, and the rest after granulation. Direct compression, Method No. 7, can also be used. The application of crospovidone in the roller compaction technology (Method No. 6) is described in the literature [650, 651].

Incorporating crospovidone prior to granulation has no adverse effect with regard to swelling, as this is reversible and – in contrast to carboxymethyl starch – the swelling effect and the disintegration time remain unchanged by wetting and drying [405].

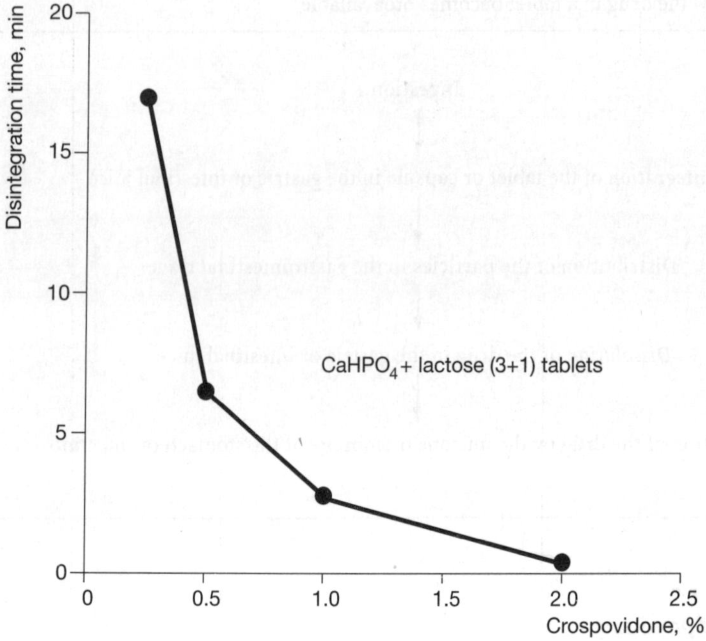

Fig. 75. Effect of the concentration of crospovidone on the disintegration time of calcium hydrogen phosphate-lactose tablets [396]

Nevertheless, adding the disintegrant after granulation makes it easier to reprocess a batch of tablets, should this become necessary [243].

It is always worth investigating the relative merits of adding crospovidone before or after granulation (Methods 3–6 in Table 132) whenever problems occur in tabletting. As shown in Table 133 for magnesium trisilicate tablets, the addition of 4% crospovidone prior to granulation reduces the friability of the tablets without noticeably changing their disintegration or hardness, compared to when it is added after granulation.

In a few cases, the inclusion of the disintegrant in the granulation mixture can provide tablets with shorter disintegration times [216]. This particularly applies when the tablet disintegrates quickly enough, but the granules do not, as when they are very hard. In such cases, it is recommended to add some of the crospovidone before granulation and some after. Such combination of the extragranular and intragranular addition was the best method to obtain the optimal release of atenolol or an other watersoluble drug from tablets [635, 640].

The solubility of the tabletting mixture (drug and/or filler) in water also has a definite influence on the effectiveness of disintegrants. These are often more effective in insoluble mixtures. Thus, for instance, calcium phosphate placebo tablets with 4% crospovidone disintegrate significantly more quickly than corresponding tablets with lactose [441].

Table 132. General tabletting methods with particular regard to the point of addition of the disintegrant

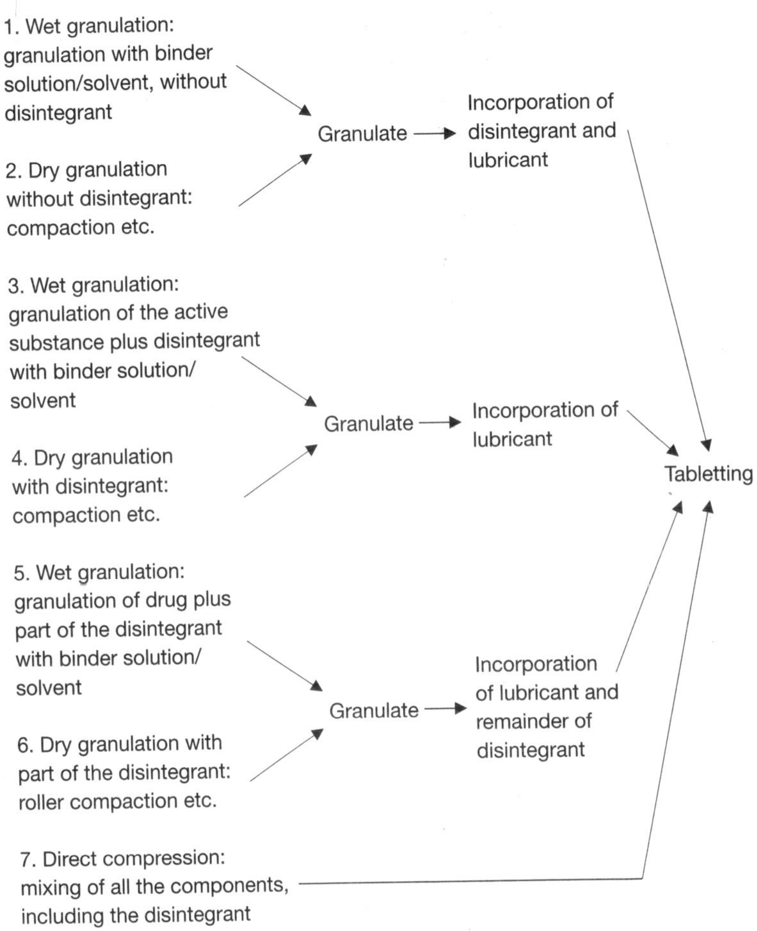

Table 133. Effect of adding 4% crospovidone before or after granulation on the properties of magnesium trisilicate tablets [397]

Parameter	Intragranular addition	Extragranular addition
Hardness	108 N	110 N
Disintegration	30 s	36 s
Friability	2.3%	1.6%

3.4.2.3
The influence of compression force on tablet hardness

The addition of crospovidone has no adverse effect on tablet hardness. The hardness often remains proportional to the compression force over a wide range [404, 390], so that tablets of high hardness and rapid disintegration can be obtained. The performance of crospovidone, starch and carboxymethyl starch in hydrochlorothiazide is compared in Fig. 76.

The compression force and the tablet hardness usually have little effect on the disintegration time of tablets that contain crospovidone. This means that it is possible to achieve short disintegration times and rapid dissolution of the active substance with good tablet hardness [393, 404]. The relationship between compression force and the disintegration time of drug-containing tablets made with crospovidone is also described in the literature [243, 390]. In Fig. 77, the curve for crospovidone is the lowest, indicating that the compression force has little effect on disintegration.

It has also been found with acetaminophen tablets that, compared with other disintegrants, the addition of 2% crospovidone gives harder tablets with a comparable, short disintegration time at a lower compression force [402]. Lactose gives tablets with similar properties [262].

Crospovidone normally improves the dissolution of a substance from the tablet. As with the disintegration time, the dissolution is usually not adversely

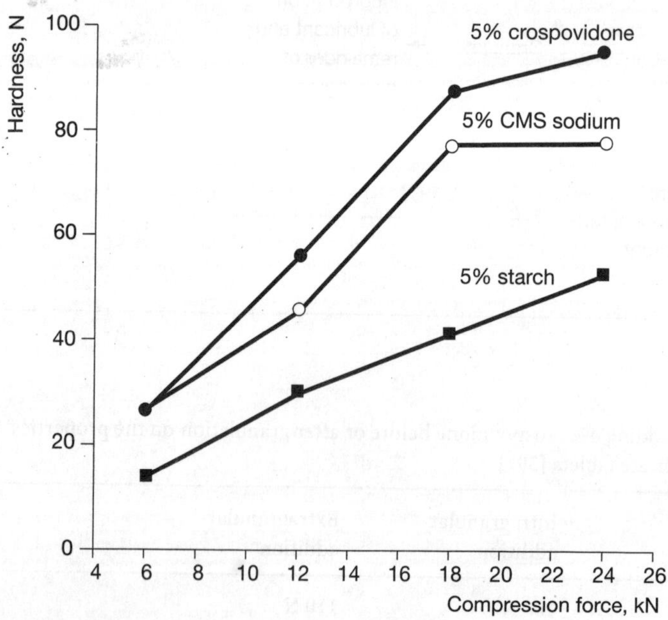

Fig. 76. Influence of compression force on the hardness of hydrochlorothiazide tablets containing 5 % of disintegrant [390]

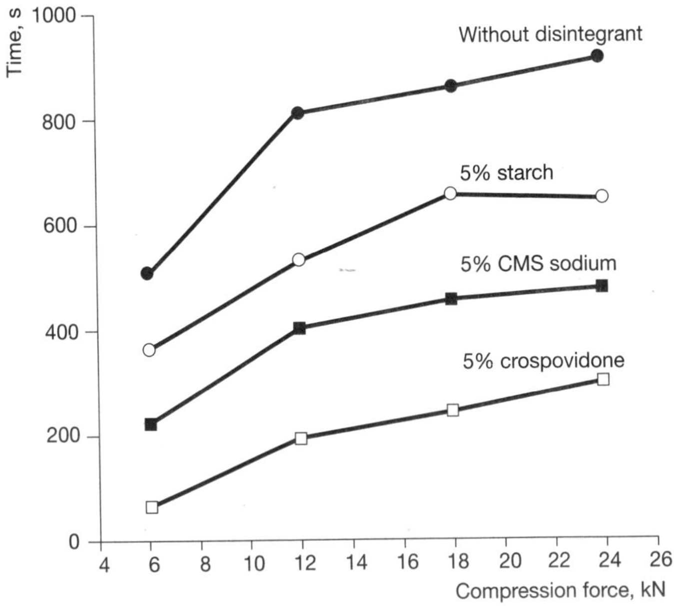

Fig. 77. Effect of compression force on the disintegration time of drug-containing tablets with different disintegrants [390]

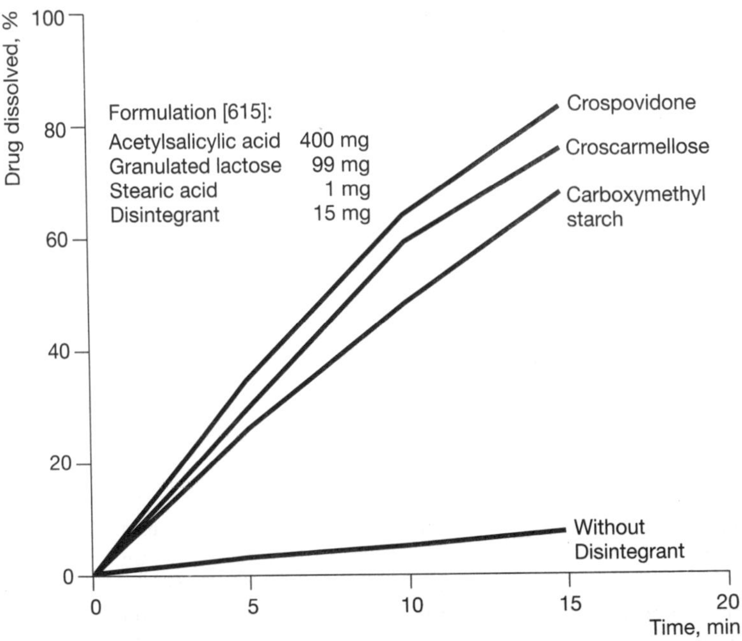

Fig. 78. Dissolution of acetylsalicylic acid tablets according to USP prepared with different disintegrants (3%)

affected over a certain compression force range. This was reported in the case of amaranth placebo tablets with 5% crospovidone. The dissolution rate of the dye was not reduced at higher compression forces [91]. Figure 78 shows the dissolution of acetylsalicylic acid tablets prepared with crospovidone, croscarmellose, carboxymethyl starch or without disintegrant. The increase of the dissolution in comparison with the tablets without disintegrant is enormous.

3.4.2.4
The influence of storage on the physical properties of tablets

Changes in the physical properties, e. g. hardness, disintegration and dissolution of tablets are a common problem. An important feature of crospovidone is that the disintegration times of tablets made with it remain largely unchanged over long periods, if they are correctly packaged. To demonstrate this, an analgesic tablet (250 mg acetylsalicylic acid + 250 mg phenacetin + 50 mg caffeine) with 5% disintegrant was stored for 12 months at room temperature. Crospovidone was the only one of the five disintegrants tested that gave tablets whose short disintegration time of 1 min did not change during storage. The disintegration times of tablets made with the other disintegrants were longer from the start and increased markedly during storage (Table 134). The hardness and friability of the tablets remained largely unchanged, regardless of the formulation. Similar results are described for the dissolution time of hydrochlorothiazide tablets [543].

Even when calcium hydrogen phosphate tablets with 2.5% crospovidone were stored for 3 months at 75% relative humidity, the rate of dissolution of the amaranth dye was increased rather than reduced [95]. Similar results were obtained with tiaramide tablets [405].

Table 137 shows the results of storing para-aminobenzoic acid tablets containing 2% crospovidone for 14 months at 30 °C [403]. Here, too, no reduction in the release of the drug was found after storage.

The packaging always has a major effect on the properties of tablets that contain crospovidone, when they are stored under humid conditions. Crospovidone is highly hygroscopic and the individual particles begin to swell when they

Table 134. The influence of storage at room temperature on the disintegration of analgesic tablets

Disintegrant (5%)	Disintegration in synthetic gastric juice After preparation	After 12 months
Crospovidone	1 min	1 min
Croscarmellose	7 min	12 min
Carmellose	22 min	46 min
Carboxymethyl starch	16 min	48 min
L-Hydroxypropyl cellulose	15 min	20 min

adsorb water (see also Section 3.4.6.2). This can have two detrimental effects. Firstly, the surface of the tablets becomes rough and unsightly, and secondly, the tablets become softer [95]. It is therefore important to always provide the tablets with moisture-proof packaging.

On the other hand, crospovidone can indirectly stabilize drugs in tablets by adsorbing water (see also Section 3.4.6.2). Water promotes degradation and other reactions, particularly in multivitamin tablets [368d].

3.4.2.5
Comparison of crospovidone with other disintegrants

As not all disintegrants function in the same manner, and as their action is not only based on swelling, they can behave somewhat differently, depending on the tablet formulation. This is why the physical methods given in Table 119 in Section 3.2.4 do not allow reliable comparison of the disintegrants used today. The same applies also to a large number of investigations using placebo tablets [e.g. 89–91, 95, 167, 191, 216, 392, 393, 396, 404, 441]. A combination of several of these methods is more likely to provide information that is relevant to practical requirements [391]. In view of the fact that the dissolution is the final quality criteria of the effect of a disintegrant in a tablet these published physical characterizations of disintegration are more of theoretical interest.

Thus, there is no ideal disintegrant for all tablets or capsules and it is necessary to compare different disintegrants in the same drug formulation (see also Figs. 69 to 71). Table 135 lists a series of publications in which disintegrant trials on drug-containing tablets or capsules are described. Unfortunately, not all the papers contain investigations into the dissolution of the drug.

Table 135. Literature on comparisons between different disintegrants

Drug	Disintegration test	Dissolution test	Literature source
Acetaminophen (paracetamol)	+	+	[402]
Acetphenetidin	+	+	[94, 392]
Acetylsalicylic acid	+	+	[239]
Acetylsalicylic acid	+	–	[398, 404]
p-Aminobenzoic acid	+	+	[403]
Amoxicillin	+	–	[519]
Ampicillin	+	–	[519]
Ascorbic acid	+	+	[239]
Cefalexin	+	–	[519]
Cefadroxil	+	–	[519]
Diazepam	+	–	[96]
Diethylenediamine sultosylate	+	+	[210]
Experimental product (Pfizer)	+	–	[243] ▶

Table 135. Continued

Drug	Disintegration test	Dissolution test	Literature source
Harpagophytum plant extract	+	–	[250]
Hydrochlorothiazide	+	+	[390, 543]
Ibuprofen	–	+	[555, 584]
Ketoconazol	+	+	[525]
Magnesium trisilicate	+	–	[397]
Prednisone	+	+	[216]
Terfenadin	+	+	[553]
Tiaramide HCl	+	–	[405]

Table 136. Comparison of disintegrants in analgesic tablets

1. Composition

I	Acetaminophen cryst.	250 mg
	Acetylsalicylic acid cryst.	250 mg
	Caffeine cryst.	50 mg
II	Povidone K 90 (dissolved in 2-propanol)	17 mg
III	Magnesium stearate	5 mg
	Disintegrant	27 mg

Granulate Mixture I with Solution II, sieve, dry and mix with III and press on a rotary tablet press.

2. Disintegration times of the tablets in synthetic gastric juice

Disintegrant	Minutes
None	> 30
Crospovidone	2
Croscarmellose	12
Carboxymethylstarch	25
L-HPC	14

As a result of examining many publications on comparisons between disintegrants in tablet or capsules formulations, it can be said in summary that crospovidone can be counted as one of the three "superdisintegrants" [216, 403, 441, 654]. This is demonstrated by the examples in Tables 136 to 138.

A further result of these publications and references is that a difference of the disintegration time of few minutes normally has not any significant influence on the dissolution of the active ingredient.

Table 137. Comparison of disintegrants in a p-aminobenzoic acid tablet before and after storage [403]

1. Composition

p-Aminobenzoic acid	1.0%
Sorbitol	48.3%
Dicalcium phosphate	48.3%
Magnesium stearate	0.5%
Disintegrant	2.0%

2. Dissolution of the drug after 15 min

Disintegrant	After manufacture	After 14 months storage at 30°C (packaged)
None	27%	34%
Crospovidone (Kollidon® CL)	78%	81%
Crospovidone (Polyplasdone® XL)	79%	82%
Croscarmellose	80%	74%
Carboxymethyl starch	68%	74%

Table 138. Comparison of disintegrants in prednisone tablets [216]

1. Composition

I	Prednisone	1.0%
	Disintegrant	4.0%
	Lactose	94.5%
II	Gelatin (dissolved in water)	0.5%

Granulate Mixture I with Solution II, dry, sieve and press into tablets.

2. Properties of the tablets

Disintegrant	Disintegration time	Dissolution (10 min)
Potato starch (20%)	215 s	65%
Crospovidone	26 s	99%
Croscarmellose	149 s	93%
Carboxymethylcellulose	424 s	45%
Carboxymethyl starch	49 s	100%

3.4.2.6
Comparison of normal and micronized crospovidone

Differences can be seen not only between the chemically different disintegrants but also between normal and micronized crospovidones, which give very different disintegration times.

Although the swelling pressure of micronized crospovidone is the same as that of the normal product, the disintegration effect depends on the size of the particles. Tablets disintegrate more rapidly if the individual particles of crospovidone are larger. This was tested in the acetaminophen-acetylsalicylic acid-caffeine tablet, whose formulation is given in Table 136, with a normal crospovidone and its micronized form not available in the market. It can be seen from the results shown in Fig. 79 that the normal crospovidone gives a much faster disintegration than the same product after micronization (more than 90 % below 50 μm).

Two different commercial crospovidone types also were compared in analgesic tablets of similar composition to that given in Table 136. Table 139 shows that the disintegration effect of normal crospovidone is many times greater than that of a commercial micronized crospovidone. There was no difference in the hardness of the tablets. The explanation for the difference is to be found in the different swelling characteristics of the two products (see Section 3.2.4).

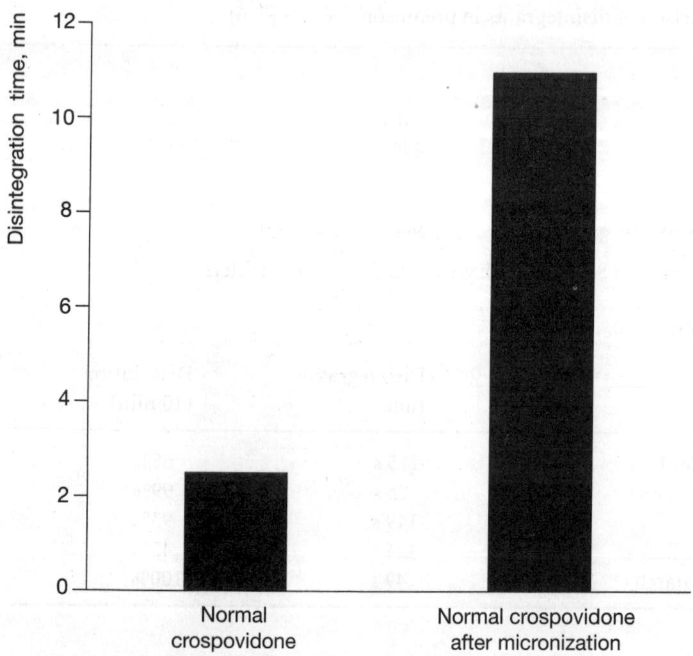

Fig. 79. Effect of the particle size of crospovidone before and after micronization on the disintegration of analgesic tablets (formulation: see Table 136)

Table 139. Comparison of commercial normal and micronized crospovidones in analgesic tablets

	Proportion in the tablet	Hardness	Disintegration time
Normal crospovidone (Kollidon® CL)	3%	63 N	2 min
	5%	60 N	1 min
Micronized crospovidone (Kollidon® CL-M)	3%	61 N	15 min
	5%	59 N	6 min

In hydrochlorothiazid tablets almost all commercial types of crospovidone were compared using soluble and insoluble fillers [662]. In the case of dicalcium phosphate as filler the disintegration times and dissolution results of the active ingredient depend strongly on the type of crospovidone used. In the case of lactose as filler no significant difference between all crospovidone types could be seen in the disintegration time of the tablet and the dissolution rate of hydrochlorothiazide.

It can be concluded that the efficacy of the use of a normal or a micronized crospovidone as disintegrant and dissolution agent depends on the formulation but usually the normal grades disintegrates faster than the micronized grades.

The particle size of the normal crospovidone grades available in the market can be considered as a compromise. Although a coarser product provides a better disintegration effect than a finer one, the latter can give tablets whose surface finish is less affected by high humidity than tablets made with a coarser crospovidone.

3.4.2.7
Coating of tablets that contain crospovidone

As tablet cores that contain crospovidone or croscarmelose swell readily in the presence of water, care must be taken when coating such tablets with aqueous solutions in the coating pan [493]. In many cases it is advisable to subcoat the cores before applying the actual sugar or film coating.

A 10% solution of copovidone in alcohol, ethyl acetate or 2-propanol has been found to give good results in subcoating. The solution is sprayed onto the prewarmed tablet cores for a short time in the same coating machine in which the final aqueous coating is to be applied (see Section 4.4.3.2).

3.4.2.8
The use of crospovidone as a disintegrant in suppositories

Crospovidone can be used as a disintegrant to increase the bioavailability not only of tablets, but also of suppositories. The dissolution rate of drugs in polyethylene glycol-based suppositories can be improved by adding 1–10% of crospovidone [211].

3.4.2.9
The use of crospovidone in fast dispersible tablets

During the last years fast dispersible tablets for the disintegration in the mouth were developed and commercialized e.g. Flash tabs®. First of all this applies to analgesic drugs. For this kind of tablets the "superdisintegrants" like crospovidone are used to obtain a disintegration within less than one minute. A typical example is ibuprofen [654, 655].

3.4.3
Improvement of the dissolution and bioavailability of insoluble drugs with crospovidone

3.4.3.1
General

As described in Section 3.4.2, crospovidone can contribute to improving the dissolution and bioavailability of a drug, as a result of its disintegrating properties. However, these properties are inadequate for a number of drug substances, as their solubility in gastric juice is poor. In such cases it is worth considering complexing them with crospovidone in the same manner as with povidone (see Section 3.2.5.1).

It is interesting to note that, although crospovidone is insoluble, it can be used in solid pharmaceutical preparations to improve the dissolution rate of an active substance. That this is not merely the result of a short-term increase in the surface area of the active substance but of the formation of a complex, can be seen in Fig. 80. Simply mixing indomethacin with crospovidone multiplies the dissolution rate of this drug substance during more than two hours. Similar results were obtained with indoprofen [439], propyphenazone [426] and prostaglandin ester [359].

Furthermore Fig. 80 shows that povidone and crospovidone increase in a comparable way the dissolution of indomethacin forming the same complex between drug and polymer. As the particle size and the swelling of these two polmers is quite different, this could explain the slight difference of dissolution.

There are a number of techniques to take advantage of this property of the crospovidone:

- Physical mixture
- Trituration (co-milling or co-grinding)
- Coevaporation after mixing a solution of the drug with crospovidone

If one of the first two techniques gives the desired result, it is always preferable to the coevaporation technique, as this requires the use of a solvent (see Figs. 80/82).

The influence of the drug/auxiliary ratio was investigated for cavain [38]. The results in Fig. 81 show clearly that more than three parts of crospovidone are

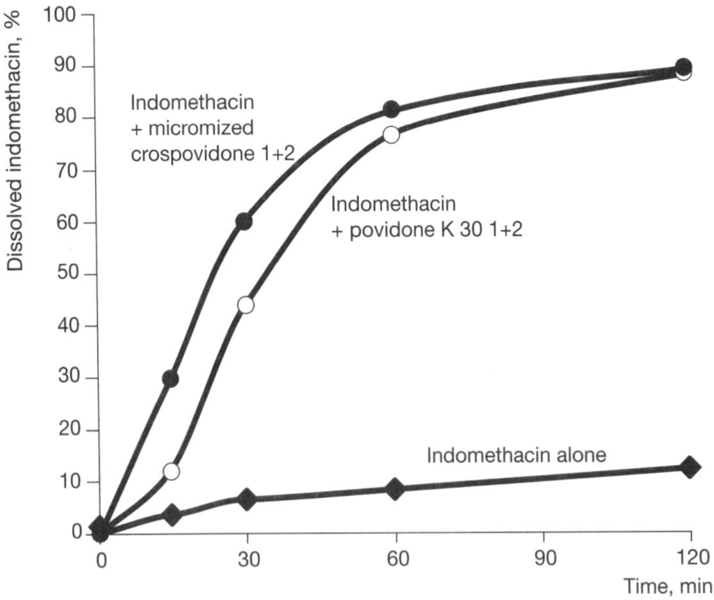

Fig. 80. Improvement of the dissolution fo indomethacin in water at 25°C mixing with crospovidone or povidone

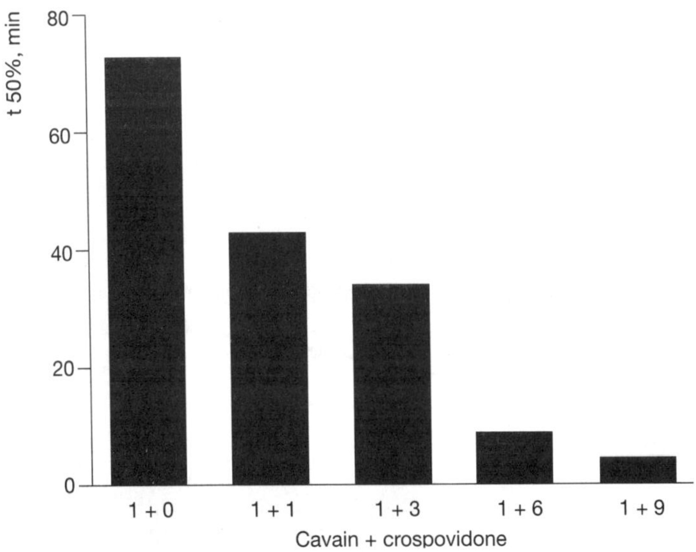

Fig. 81. Influence of the proportion of crospovidone on the dissolution time (t 50 %) of cavain [38]

required for one part of this drug to accelerate its dissolution by a worthwhile amount. The best results with other drugs are also obtained with an excess of the polymer. In the case of cavain, the optimum ratio is between 1 + 3 and 1 + 6.

3.4.3.2
Triturations

The factor by which the dissolution of an active substance is increased by triturating it with crospovidone usually lies between 2 and 10 but can exceed 10. This is shown in Fig. 82 for medroxyprogesterone acetate tablets, in which a six-fold excess of crospovidone improves the dissolution rate by a factor of 5, compared with that of tablets without this excipient. But in the some cases such factor of 5 already can be achieved by the ratio 1 + 2 (see Figs. 80 and 83).

The optimum time of trituration must be determined individually for each active substance. Factors that must be taken into consideration include the dissolution rate, bioavailability, chemical and physical stability of the drug, and the costs. Usually one hour is adequate.

Recent trials have shown that in triturations with certain drugs, reducing the size of the crospovidone particles improves the dissolution rate and bioavailability. One possible reason is the increase of the specific surface area achieved, for example, by micronization (see Section 3.2.3.1). However, the absolute value of the

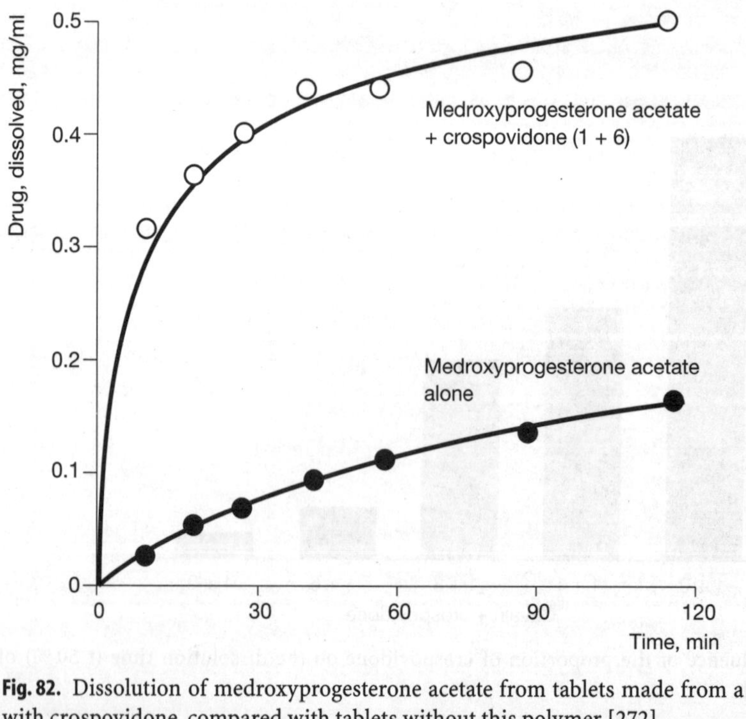

Fig. 82. Dissolution of medroxyprogesterone acetate from tablets made from a trituration with crospovidone, compared with tablets without this polymer [272]

Table 140. Drugs whose dissolution rate is increased by trituration or physical mixing with crospovidone

Drug	Increased dissolution	Physical state	Stability of the state	Literature source
Ansamycin	+	amorphous	stable	[272]
Atenolol	+	partly amorphous	n.d.	[613]
Carbamazepin	+	cryst.	n.d.	[565]
Diacerein	+	n.d.	n.d.	[364, 365]
Diacetyl-midecamycin	n.d.	amorphous	stable	[432]
Diltiazem	+	n.d.	n.d.	[365]
Etoposide	+	n.d.	n.d.	[139]
Furosemide	+	amorphous	stable	[617]
Griseofulvin	+	n.d.	n.d.	[364, 365, 440 b]
Indomethacin	+	n.d.	n.d.	[365]
Indoprofen	+	n.d.	n.d	[439, 440 b]
Medroxypro-gesterone acetate	+	amorphous	stable	[272, 440]
Megestrol acetate	+	n.d.	n.d.	[364, 365]
Nicergoline	+	n.d.	n.d.	[365]
Piroxicam	+	n.d.	n.d.	[365]
Uracil	+	amorphous	n.d.	[380]

n.d. = not determined

specific surface area appears to play only a subordinate role, as normal crospovidone is more effective than one of the micronized types in individual cases, although the latter had twice the surface area. On the other hand, it only develops half the swelling force.

All the active substances investigated so far were converted to the amorphous form by trituration with crospovidone, and this always remained stable in the few trials that have been conducted so far (Table 140). Stability results are available for a much larger number of drugs in coevaporates with crospovidone (Table 141). As all the drugs tested in coevaporates were found to have very good physical stability of their amorphous state, the same can be assumed for triturations. This correlates with similar results obtained with povidone (see Section 2.4.3.2).

Table 140 contains a selection of literature references of drugs with which triturations with crospovidone have been prepared.

3.4.3.3
Coevaporates

The technique of coevaporation has been adopted for crospovidone from povidone. The earliest papers were published in 1978 [36]. The drug is dissolved in a suitable solvent, crospovidone is wetted with this solution, and the solvent is then evaporated. A disadvantage of this technique, compared with trituration, is that it requires an organic solvent.

The effect on dissolution of coevaporating furosemide is shown in Fig. 83. The dissolution rate increases by a factor of 5–10 for a drug:crospovidone ratio of 1:2 compared with that for furosemide alone and the ground mixture 1:2.

More papers have been published on coevaporates of drugs with crospovidone than on triturations. In particular, the state (crystalline/amorphous) of the active substance and its stability have been investigated much more frequently (Table 141). In no case was a return to the crystalline form reported. The chemical stability of indomethacin in a coevaporate has been reported. The stability was found to be good in an accelerated test [401]. As it has also been found to be good in a large number of drug coprecipitates with povidone, the same can be assumed with a high degree of certainty for coevaporates with crospovidone.

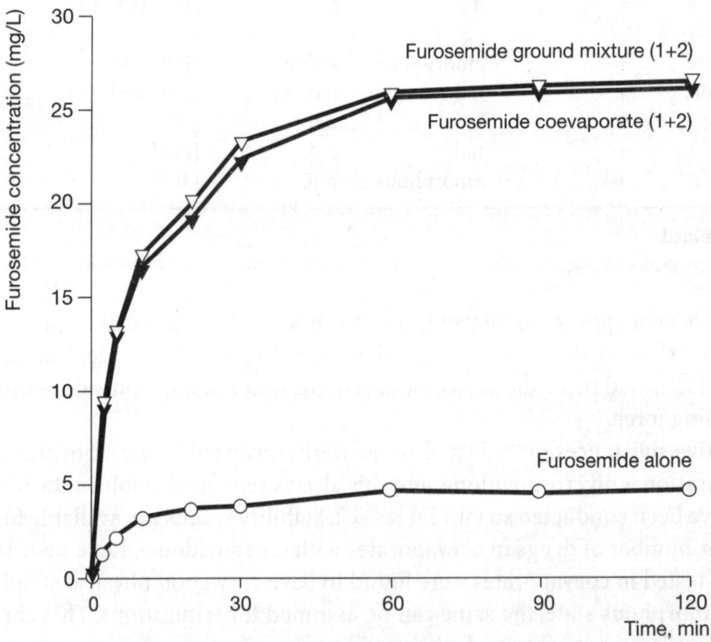

Fig. 83. Dissolution of furosemide from preparations with crospovidone [617]

Table 141. Active substances whose dissolution rate is improved by coevaporation with crospovidone

Drug	Increased dissolution	Physical state	Stability of the state	Literature source
Carbamazepin	+	cryst.	n.d.	[565]
Cavain	+	amorphous	stable	[36, 38]
Dexamethasone	+	amorphous	n.d.	[457]
Ethyl biscoum-acetate	+	amorphous	stable	[36]
Flufenamic acid	+	amorphous	n.d.	[207]
Furosemide	+	amorphous	stable	[486, 617]
Griseofulvin	+	amorphous	stable	[36, 232]
Hexobarbital	+	amorphous	n.d.	[36, 37]
Indomethacin	+	amorphous	stable	[222, 273]
Itraconazole	+	amorphous	n.d.	[642]
Medroxypro-gesterone acetate	+	amorphous	n.d.	[272, 440]
Megestrol acetate	+	n.d.	n.d.	[271]
Nifedipine	+	n.d.	n.d.	[240c, 364]
Nimodipine	+	n.d.	n.d.	[240c, 364]
Nitrendipin	+	n.d.	n.d.	[240c]
Phenprocoumon	+	amorphous	stable	[36]
Phenytoin	+	amorphous	stable	[36]
Propyphenazone	+	n.d.	n.d.	[426]
Prostaglandin ester	+	n.d.	n.d.	[359]
Tolbutamide	+	amorphous	stable	[36]

n.d. = not determined

3.4.3.4
Bioavailability

Unfortunately, the many publications listed in Tables 140 and 141 contain only a few drugs whose bioavailability has been tested in animals or in man. It has been significantly higher for all the drugs tested (ansamycin [272], hexobarbital [37], medroxyprogesterone acetate [272, 440 b], megestrol acetate [271]). This is shown more clearly in Fig. 84 for megestrol acetate tablets, which were formulated with a 1 +3 drug-crospovidone coevaporate. The bioavailability from coevaporate tablets after a single administration in dogs was about twice as high as from tablets with micronized megestrol acetate alone.

In principle, an improvement in the dissolution rate and bioavailability of all the drugs, whose dissolution and bioavailability can be accelerated with povidone (Section 2.4.3) can also be expected if they are coevaporated or triturated with crospovidone. This may be expected, as the effect of increasing the surface area by

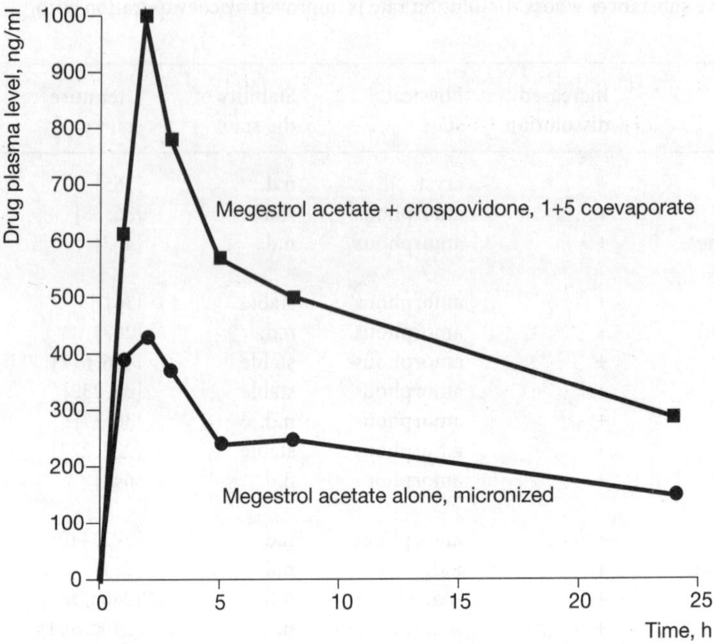

Fig. 84. Bioavailability in dogs of megestrol acetate from tablets [271]

reducing the size of the crystals, or even converting the active substance to an amorphous form [38, 207], and the effect of complexation are comparable [192].

3.4.4 Micronized crospovidone of low bulk density as a stabilizer for oral and topical suspensions

3.4.4.1 *General*

From a physical point of view, suspensions are usually unstable systems, as the solid phase almost always tends to form a sediment. One of the most important aims with this type of dosage form must therefore be to prevent sedimentation. As this ideal condition can usually not be achieved, it is at least attempted to reduce the sedimentation rate and, above all, to make any sediment easy to redisperse. A number of auxiliaries are used in pharmaceutical technology to achieve this. They include thickeners, hydrophilic polymers, sugars and sugar alcohols, surfactants and electrolytes [296]. In spite of its insolubility, crospovidone can be classed as a hydrophilic polymer.

The function of these polymers is governed mainly by Stokes' law (Table 142), which states that the rate of sedimentation is proportional to the square of the

Table 142. Stokes' law

$$\text{Sedimentation rate, cm/s} = \frac{2\,r^2\,(d_1 - d_2)\,g}{9\,\eta}$$

η = viscosity of the suspension
r = radius of the particles
d_1 = density of the suspended phase
d_2 = density of the continuous phase
g = gravity

radius of the suspended particles and the difference in density between them and the continuous phase, and inversely proportional to the viscosity.

The effect of low-density micronized crospovidone (e.g. Kollidon® CL-M) in stabilizing suspensions can also be partly explained in terms of Stokes' law. Its particle size is very fine (see Section 3.2.2), its bulk density low and its density in water also low as a result of swelling. The product differs in these properties from the coarser products and other micronized types which have a higher bulk density with a similar swelling volume, and make it useful as an auxiliary for oral and topical suspensions for reducing sedimentation and improving redispersibility [98]. The same applies, whether the commercial product is a suspension or a dry syrup, or instant granules from which the patient prepares an oral suspension.

When micronized crospovidone of low bulk density is used in such suspensions, it is found beneficial in practice to combine it with other auxiliaries such as sodium citrate as an electrolyte, sugar, poloxamer or povidone, to increase the sediment volume. In the example given in Section 2.4.6.2 (Fig. 55), this is done by adding povidone K 90. A suspension of 7.5% of low-density micronized crospovidone with 5% povidone K 90 showed no further sedimentation after a 24-hour test.

Even better results were obtained with drug formulations, the redispersibility being at least as important as the sediment volume.

3.4.4.2
Concentrations, viscosity

According to the current knowledge the usual concentrations of low-density micronized crospovidone are 5–10% in suspensions.

In individual cases, the concentration may be lower or higher. At these usual concentrations, the viscosity evidently does not play a role in preventing sedimentation, as it is relatively low.

To determine the importance of viscosity in suspensions containing micronized crospovidone, the viscosity of an amoxicillin dry syrup (Table 143) was measured at different concentrations. Figure 85 shows that the viscosity hardly changes over

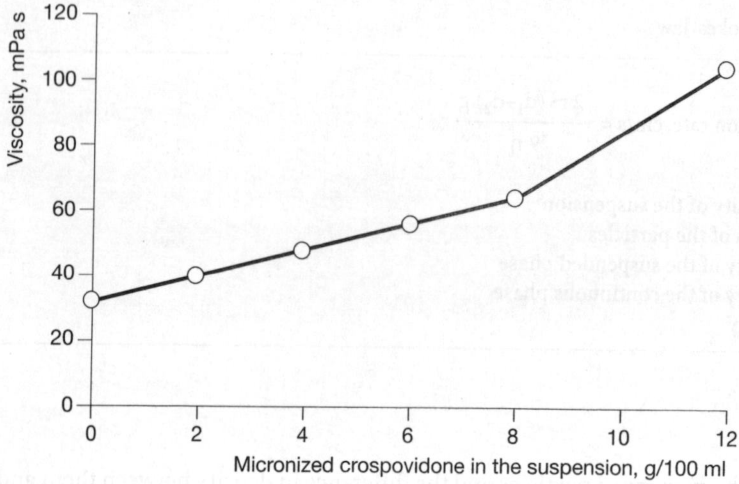

Fig. 85. Influence of the concentration of micronized crospovidone of low bulk density on the viscosity of an amoxicillin suspension (Table 143)

a range of 0–8% crospovidone. However, the relative sediment volume increased greatly, as can be seen from Fig. 86.

3.4.4.3
Examples of applications

Dry syrups and instant granules are more important these days than finished suspensions, as the active ingredient is more stable in these dry products, and the physical stability requirements of the suspension, as the actual administration form, are not so critical. Because of their stability, dry syrups are often used as the dosage form for antibiotics. Instant granules are widely used for antacids, because of the possibility of microbial contamination with finished suspensions, for vitamins (plus minerals) for stability reasons, and for analgesics.

An antibiotic dry syrup formulation is shown in Table 143 as an application of micronized crospovidone of low bulk density. The formulation has been developed in the laboratory for two different drugs, so that it can be regarded as a typical guide formulation. It contains citric acid, to adjust the pH to 4.9, to optimize the chemical stability of the drug, ampicillin trihydrate or amoxicillin trihydrate.

The optimum quantity of 6% crospovidone in the formulation in Table 143 was determined from the relative sediment volume. Figure 86 shows that, at this concentration, no further sedimentation takes place after 24 hours. With lower quantities of micronized crospovidone, a sediment was clearly visible.

The laboratory formulation in Table 144 provides an example of the use in acetaminophen instant granules, e.g. for children [296]. In this formulation, micronized crospovidone has two additional functions: it masks the bitter taste of acetaminophen almost completely, and it guarantees the release of the active sub-

Table 143. Antibiotic dry syrup with micronized crospovidone for children [615]

Formulation (sales product):	
Ampicillin trihydrate or amoxicillin trihydrate	5.0 g
Sodium citrate	5.0 g
Citric acid	2.1 g
Sodium gluconate	5.0 g
Sorbitol	40.0 g
Micronized crospovidone of low bulk density	6.0 g
Orange flavour	1.5 g
Lemon flavour	0.5 g
Saccharin sodium	0.4 g

Preparation of the suspension (dosage form with 250 mg active ingredient/5 ml): shake 66 g of the powder mixture with water (total volume 100 ml).

Sedimentation is very slow and the sediment is very easy to redisperse by shaking, even after several weeks.

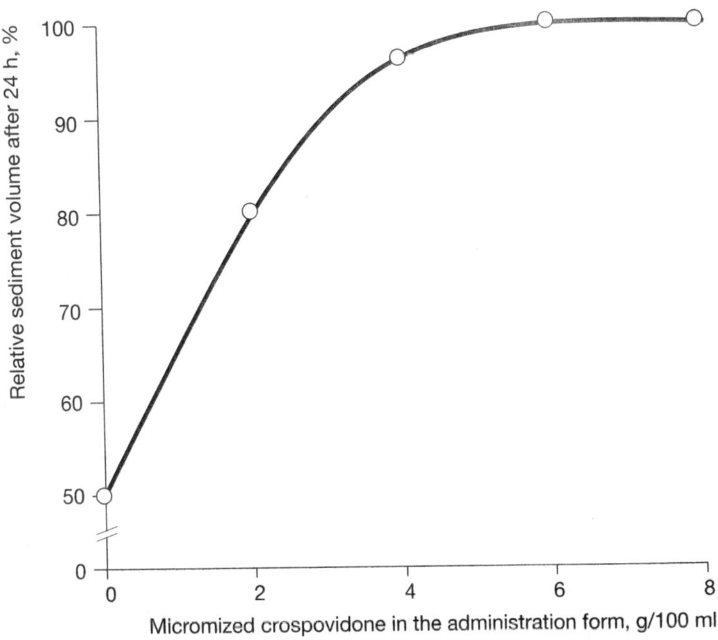

Fig. 86. Effect of the concentration of micronized crospovidone of low bulk density on the sediment volume of an amoxicillin suspension (Table 143)

Table 144. Acetaminophen instant granules [615]

1. Formulation (sales form):

I	Acetaminophen powder (< 100 μm)	50 g
	Sugar (< 100 μm)	128 g
	Micronized crospovidone of low bulk density	50 g
	Aspartame	7 g
	Orange flavour	5 g
	Strawberry flavour	5 g
II	Povidone K 30	12 g
	Ethanol 96%	75 g

Granulate Mixture I with Solution II and sieve.

2. Manufacture and properties of the suspension (administration form):
Stir 1.3 or 2.6 g of granules (= 250 or 500 mg of acetaminophen) into a glass of water. The milky suspension tastes sweet and fruity instead of bitter. No sedimentation is observed within two hours.

3. Dissolution of the active substance:
In the USP test, 94% of the active ingredient is dissolved within 5 minutes at pH 5.8.

4. Chemical stability:
In an accelerated test (2 months at 40 °C), no loss of acetaminophen was observed in the sales product.

stance, possibly by forming a complex with it, as does povidone [154]. The concentration of crospovidone in the suspension of these acetaminophen instant granules is well below 1% and therefore significantly lower than in dry syrups, as, in this case, the suspension only needs to be stabilized for a very short time. The chemical stability of the sales product, which can be packaged in individual sachets, was very good in an accelerated test.

In an azithromycin dry syrup micronized crospovidone not only stabilizes the suspension physically but also masks the bitter taste of the drug substance [615]. The formulation given in Table 145 was also developed on a laboratory scale and demonstrates the use of micronized crospovidone in an antiacid dry syrup from which a suspension is prepared as the administration form.

Again, the quantity of micronized crospovidone was determined from the relative sediment volume. As is evident from Fig. 87, no sedimentation was observed above a crospovidone concentration of 9% in the final suspension (= 29 g crospovidone in the sales product). After several weeks, it was still very easy to redisperse the suspension with a few rocking movements.

Table 145. Antiacid dry syrup [615]

1. Formulation (sales form):

I	Aluminium hydroxide dried gel (Giulini)	25.0 g
	Magnesium carbonate basic	25.0 g
	Micronized crospovidone of low bulk density	29.0 g
	Sorbitol	25.6 g
	Orange flavour	5.0 g
II	Povidone K 30	10.0 g
	Coconut flavour	0.4 g
	Banana flavour	0.5 g
	Saccharin sodium	0.1 g
	Water	ca. 36 ml

Granulate Mixture I with Solution II, sieve and dry.

2. Administration form:
Shake 120 g of the granulate with 200 ml of water.

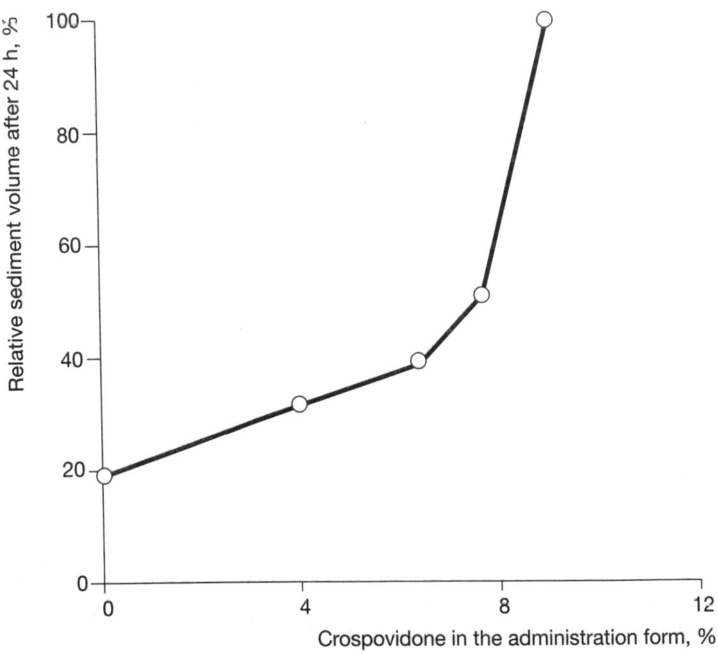

Fig. 87. Influence of the concentration of micronized crospovidone of low bulk density on the relative sediment volume of the antiacid suspension described in Table 141 [296]

3.4.5
Micronized crospovidone as an active substance

As early as 1968, a patent was granted for the use of insoluble polyvinyl pyrrolidone as an active substance for treating certain stomach and intestinal disorders [125]. Pharmaceutical products containing micronized crospovidone as an active substance have been sold in France since the 70s on the basis of the results in a series of publications [443–454]. They contain 2g of crospovidone per dose, which, in one case, is combined with karaya gum as a further active substance. The functions and medical indications listed in Table 146 are to be found in the clinical literature and with the pharmaceutical products. This application of micronized crospovidone is based on the local effect on the mucous membrane, as opposed to a systemic effect, as it is insoluble and therefore not absorbed. This is why practically no side-effects are listed.

The preferred dosage forms are "instant drink tablets" for suspension in a glass of water, instant granules, and ready suspensions. These dosage forms make it possible both for adults and children to take the large quantity of active substance without problems.

Table 147 gives a guide formulation developed in the laboratory for effervescent tablets for children, containing 1 g of micronized crospovidone as the active ingredient. No problems are to be expected with the chemical stability of this formulation. However, moisture-proof packaging is recommended, to stabilize the physical properties of the tablets for the duration of their intended shelf-life.

In another formulation for a water-dispersible tablet based on 74% crospovidone, containing as auxiliaries, microcrystalline cellulose, corn starch, silicon dioxide, talc etc. [615], it was possible to confirm that the compression force and

Table 146. Properties, functions and indications of crospovidone as an active substance against gastrointestinal complaints

1. Functions and properties [444, 447, 449, 452]
- Formation of a protective layer on the mucous membranes
- Adsorption of gas
- Adsorption of water
- Swellability
- Complexation of toxins of microbial origin
- X-ray transparency

2. Medical indications (papers on clinical trials)
- Diarrhoea, dyspepsia, meteorism and other functional colopathy [125, 443, 444, 446 b, 447, 450–452, 605]
- Colitis from antibiotics [125, 443–446, 448, 453, 454]
- Gastritis [125, 451]
- Gastroduodenal ulcers [125]
- Hiatus hernia with reflux oesophagitis [125, 451]

Table 147. Formulation of crospovidone effervescent tablets (lab scale) [615]

1. Formulation

I	Crospovidone, micronized	1000 g
	Citric acid	150 g
	Aerosil® 200	25 g
II	Sucrose, crystalline	100 g
	Saccharin sodium	1 g
	Water	q. s.
III	Sodium bicarbonate	125 g
	Flavour	65 g
	Magnesium stearate	5 g

Granulate mixture I with solution II, pass through a 0.8-mm sieve, dry, mix with III and press into tablets on a rotary tablet press with a medium compression force.

2. Tablet properties:

Diameter	20 mm
Weight	1590 mg
Hardness	111 N
Disintegration in water	1 min
Friability	0.4 %

Table 148. Formulation of an antidiarrhoeal suspension of micronized crospovidone [615]

Micronized crospovidone (low bulk density)	20 g
Sorbitol, crystalline	10 g
Povidone K 90	2 g
Preservatives and Flavours	q. s.
Water	ad 100 ml

Dissolve sorbitol, povidone K 90, the preservatives and flavours in water, add crospovidone and homogenize by shaking.

the hardness of the tablets are directly proportional (compression curve see Fig. 88).

To produce an antidiarrhoeal suspension micronized low-density crospovidone should be used as active ingredient because its sedimentation properties are much better (see chapter 3.4.4). In the typical example given in Table 148 almost no sedimentation was observed after 4 weeks and the redispersibility is very easy.

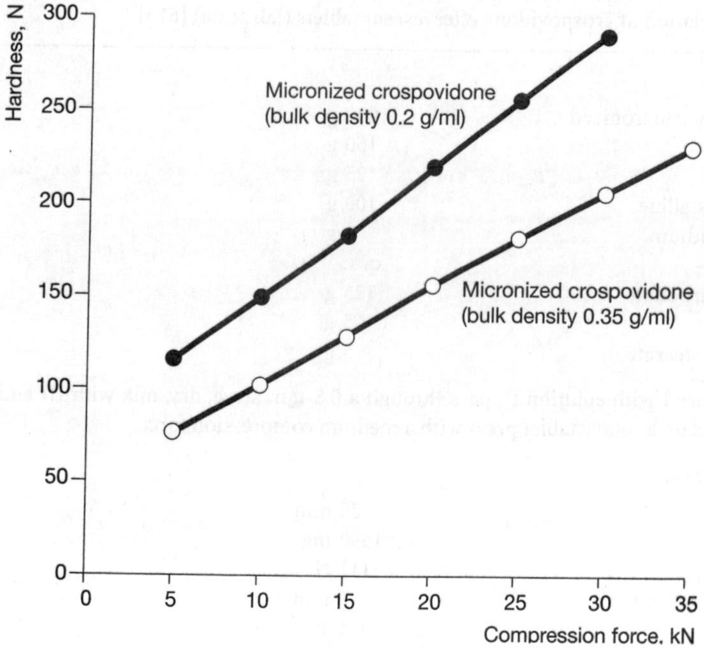

Fig. 88. Compression force/hardness curve for a water-dispersible tablet with 74% of micronzed crospovidone

3.4.6
Miscellaneous applications

3.4.6.1
Filtration aid

Because of its ability to form complexes with many chemical substances (see Section 3.2.5) and its large surface area in the swollen state, normal crospovidone is a good filtration auxiliary. It is particularly useful for selectively binding polyphenols, e.g. tannins in the form of an insoluble complex. As in the clarification of beer and wine, this feature can be used in the preparation of galenical products, particularly tinctures, aqueous and alcoholic extracts and medical wines, to extend their long-term stability by preventing precipitation.

In practice, it is best to add the crospovidone to the preparation to be purified as an aqueous slurry or as a powder. This is stirred into the preparation and then filtered off again. As an alternative, crospovidone can be used in a filtration bed, though it must be checked whether the duration of contact with the polyphenols to be bound is adequate.

3.4.6.2
Stabilization of active ingredients

As with povidone, crospovidone can also be used to stabilize drugs in pharmaceutical products. A typical example is the formulation for multivitamin drink granules [368c]. This formulation was prepared in the laboratory, and the stability of the vitamins was found to be excellent (Table 149 and 150).

Should a fluidized bed granulator not be available for the manufacture of this formulation, it is recommended not to granulate the vitamin A, B_{12}, D and E dry powders with the other ingredients but to add them to the finished granules.

The stabilization effect on the vitamins was particularly noticeable with vitamin B1, calcium D-pantothenate and ascorbic acid in an accelerated test (Table 150). For this test, the formulation in Table 149 was produced in the laboratory once with, and once without crospovidone and stored at 30°C/70% relative humidity or in sealed containers at 40°C.

Table 149. Multivitamin drink granules [368c]

1. Formulation

I	Vitamin A/D dry powder CWD	19.0 g
	Thiamine mononitrate	2.6 g
	Riboflavin	3.3 g
	Nicotinamide	11.0 g
	Pyridoxine hydrochloride	2.2 g
	Cyanocobalamin gelatin-coated 0.1%	6.6 g
	Ascorbic acid powder	115.0 g
	Tocopherol acetate dry powder SD 50	21.0 g
	Sucrose, ground	2000.0 g
	Micronized crospovidone	500.0 g
	Orange flavour	100.0 g
	Calcium D-pantothenate	150.0 g
II	Copovidone	200.0 g
	Ethanol 96%	700 ml

Granulate Mixture I with Solution II in a fluidized bed granulator. If possible, the granules should be packaged under nitrogen.

2. Vitamin loss after 12 months at 23 °C (HPLC):

Vitamin A	below 5 %
Vitamin D	below 5 %
Vitamin B_1, B_6, B_{12}	below 5 %
Calcium pantothenate	not tested
Nicotinamide	below 5 %
Ascorbic acid	6 %
Vitamin E	below 5 %

Table 150. Stabilization of vitamins in multivitamin drink granules with micronized crospovidone (Table 149)

A: Vitamin loss at 30°C/70% relative humidity

	2 months	3 months	5 months
Thiamine:			
Without crospovidone	11%	16%	26%
With crospovidone	1%	7%	10%
Ascorbic acid:			
Without crospovidone	18%	40%	49%
With crospovidone	2%	13%	19%
Calcium D-pantothenate:			
Without crospovidone	8%	21%	50%
With crospovidone	10%	10%	15%

B: Vitamin loss at 40 °C, airtight containers

	2 months	3 months
Thiamine:		
Without crospovidone	1%	7%
With crospovidone	0%	1%
Ascorbic acid:		
Without crospovidone	19%	18%
With crospovidone	3%	2%

The stabilized vitamins are sensitive against hydrolisis and chemical interactions with other vitamins. Similar to povidone [569] the stabilization effect of crospovidone could be described as desiccant action.

4 Vinylpyrrolidone-vinyl acetate copolymer (Copovidone)

4.1
Structure, synonyms

Copovidone is manufactured by free-radical polymerization of 6 parts of vinylpyrrolidone and 4 parts of vinyl acetate in 2-propanol according to the cGMP regulations. A water-soluble copolymer with a chain structure is obtained (Fig. 89).

Two commercial products of the vinylpyrrolidone-vinyl acetate copolymer are available in the market having the pharmaceutical quality required by the Pharmacopoeias. Table 151 mentions the tradenames and producers of these copovidone products.

In contrast to povidone described in Chapter 2 the numbers in the tradenames are not the K-value which characterizes the molecular weight. There is only one type of copovidone in the market having a K-value of the same order of magni-

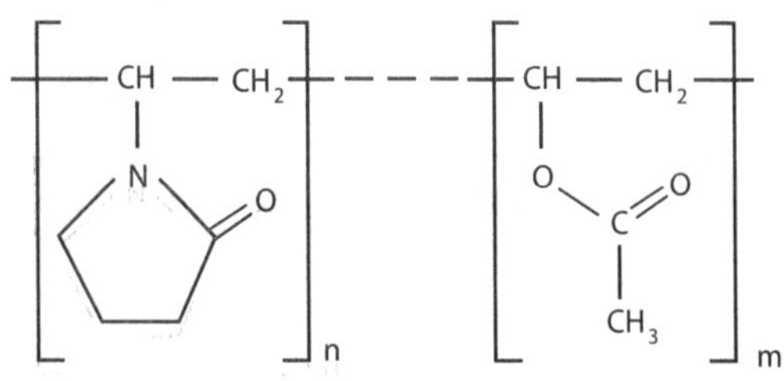

$$Mr = (111.1)_n \times (86.1)_m$$

Fig. 89. Structural formula of copovidone

Table 151. Vinylpyrrolidone-vinyl acetate copolymer 6+4 of pharmaceutical quality (= copovidone) in the market

Tradename	Manufacturer
Kollidon® VA 64	BASF (Germany)
Plasdone® S-630	ISP (USA)

Table 152. Official names and abbreviations for the vinylpyrrolidone-vinyl acetate copolymer 6 + 4

Name/abbreviation	Source
Copovidone, Copovidonum	Ph.Eur. 5, USP-NF (draft 2002)
Copolyvidone	JPE 1993
Copovidon	Deutsches Arzneibuch 1997
PVP-VAc-Copolymer	Literature

In the following, the name "copovidone" is used.

tude as that of povidone K 30 (see Table 153). The K-value is also used as a measure of the average molecular weight here (Section 4.2.3).

The CAS number of the vinylpyrrolidone-vinyl acetate copolymer 6+4 is 25086-89-9. It has the synonyms and abreviations given in Table 152.

4.2 Product properties

4.2.1 Description, specifications, pharmacopoeias

4.2.1.1 *Description*

Copovidone is a product of pharmaceutical purity. It is a white or yellowish-white spray-dried powder that has a relatively fine particle size and good flow properties. It has a typical slight odour and a faint taste in aqueous solutions.

4.2.1.2 *Pharmacopoeial requirements*

Copovidone fulfills the requirements of the "Copovidone"and "Copolyvidone" monographs in the current versions of the European Pharmacopeia (Ph.Eur. 5) and Japanese Pharmaceutical Excipients (JPE 1993). It also corresponds to the USP-NF draft monograph "Copovidone" published 2002 [652]. The current pharmacopoeial specifications are listed in Table 153. Several of the parameters are not included in the monographs but are general requirements of the pharmacopoeias.

As an alternative to the iodometric titration given in the pharmacopoeias, the monomers vinylpyrrolidone and vinyl acetate can be determined by HPLC (see Section 2.3.3.2 or 4.3.2.2). The two commercial products mentioned in Table 151 fulfill the requirement of max. 10 ppm of each monomer. The microbial status can

Table 153. Requirements of the pharmacopoeias for copovidone

Colour (10% in water):	Not darker than BY5, B5, R5
Clarity (10% in water):	Not more opalescent than reference III
Relative viscosity (1% in water):	1.178–1.255
K-value (nominally/stated 28):	25.2–30.8
Sum of monomers, iodometric:	≤ 0.1%
Loss on drying:	≤ 5%
Nitrogen:	7.0–8.0%
Saponification value:	230–270
Sulfated ash:	≤ 0.1%
Heavy metals:	≤ 10 ppm
pH (10% in water):	3–7
Peroxides (calculated as H_2O_2):	≤ 400 ppm
Hydrazine:	≤ 1 ppm
Acetaldehyde (enzymatic 2.3.3.3):	≤ 500 ppm
Polymerized vinyl acetate	35.3–42.0%
2-Pyrrolidone (see also Section 2.3.3.2)	≤ 0.5%
Residual solvents (2-propanol* and acetic acid**)	≤ 0.5%
Organic volatile impurities (USP)	Passes test
Microbial status (see Table 154)	Passes test

* Method see Section 2.3.3.5
** Method see Section 4.3.2.4

Table 154. Microbial purity requirements (Ph.Eur. 5, 5.1.4, Category 2 + 3A)

- Max. 10^2 aerobic bacteria and fungi/g
- No escherichia coli/g
- Max. 10^1 enterobacteria and other gramnegative bacteria/g
- No pseudomonas aeruginosa/g
- No staphylococcus aureus/g

be tested by Ph.Eur. methods 2.6.12 and 2.6.13. The limits are also given in Ph.Eur. (Table 154).

Copovidone meets the ICH requirements on residual solvents according to Ph.Eur. 5, chapter 5.4: Only Class 3 solvents (2-propanol, acetic acid) are likely to be present (<0.5%).

4.2.2 Solubility

Because of the ratio of vinylpyrrolidone to vinyl acetate in copovidone is almost as universally soluble as povidone. It dissolves in extremely hydrophilic liquids such as water as well as in more hydrophobic solvents such as butanol.

Table 155. Solubility of copovidone

More than 10% in:	Less than 1% in:
Water	Diethyl ether
Methanol	Pentane
Ethanol	Cyclohexane
n-Propanol	Liquid paraffin
2-Propanol	
n-Butanol	
Chloroform	
Methylene cloride	
Polyethylene glycol 400	
Propylene glycol	
1,4-Butanediol	
Glycerol	

Although nowadays the use of organic solvents such as methylene chloride or chloroform is largely avoided in the production of finished drugs, most pharmaceutical companies still use small quantities of ethanol, 2-propanol, propylene glycol or low-molecular polyethylene glycol copovidone is soluble in practically all proportions in these solvents and in water. Above a certain concentration, the viscosity of the solutions increases (see Section 4.2.3.1).

Table 155 lists a large number of solvents in which copovidone dissolves in concentrations of more than 10% or less than 1%.

The dissolution behaviour and rate are typical for a polymer. It is recommended to add the powder slowly and in small portions to the solvent, which should be vigorously stirred. This ensures that copovidone dissolves rapidly without forming lumps. Lumps are relatively slow to dissolve.

4.2.3 Viscosity, K-value, molecular weight

4.2.3.1 Viscosity

The viscosity of copovidone in water depends on its average molecular weight. This can therefore be calculated from the viscosity, to give the viscosity average of the molecular weight (see Section 4.2.3.3). Figure 90 shows the viscosity of solutions in water and in 2-propanol as a function of their concentration. The measurements were done in a capillary viscosimeter. It can be seen that solutions of about 10% have a low viscosity, which is an advantage in practice.

The viscosity of solutions of concentrations up to 10% hardly changes between 20°C and 40°C. The temperature only affects the viscosity of solutions of higher

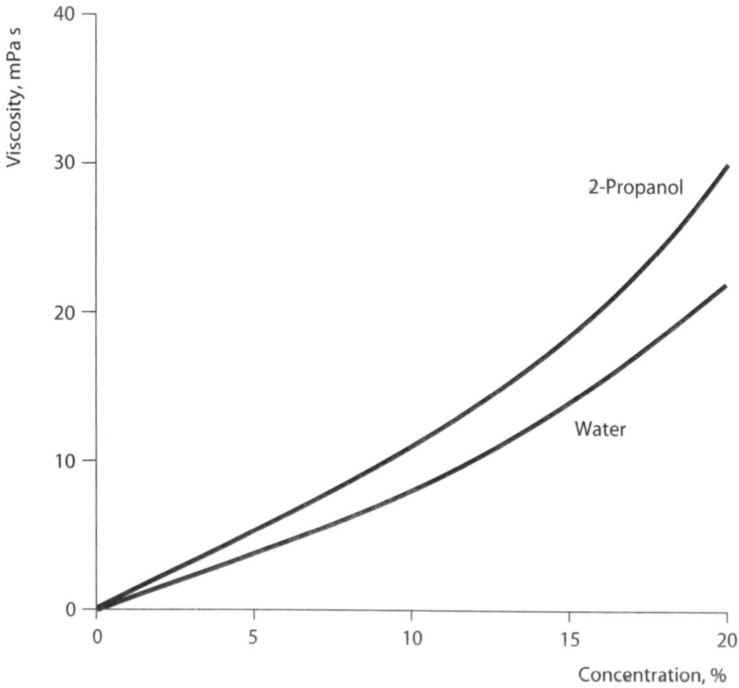

Fig. 90. The viscosity of copovidone solutions in water and 2-propanol as a function of concentration (Ubbelohde capillary viscometer, 25°C)

concentration. The viscosity of a 20% aqueous solution of copovidone remains much the same over a wide range of pH. If strongly acid or alkaline solutions are left to stand for a long time, the vinyl acetate may become saponified to some extent and the viscosity may change.

4.2.3.2
K-value

The average molecular weight of povidone and copovidone is expressed in terms of the K-value, in accordance with the Pharmacopoeias that apply in Europe and the USA [13]. It is calculated from the relative viscosity in water. The same methods can be applied to copovidone, and they give K-values between the limits given in Section 4.2.1.2. They are based on the relative viscosity of a 1% solution in water at 25°C. The relationship between the K-value and the relative viscosity is shown in Fig. 91. The curve was obtained using the method of determination and calculation described in Section 2.3.2.1.

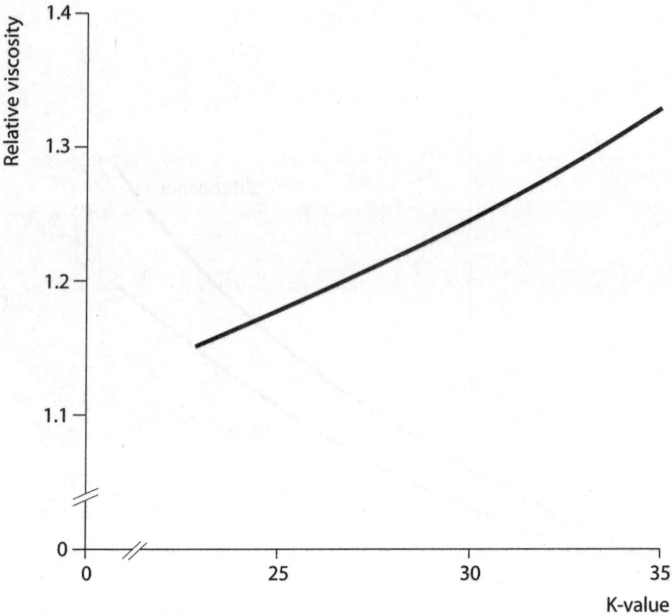

Fig. 91. Relationship between the relative viscosity (1% in water) and the K-value over a range of 23–35 [13]

4.2.3.3 *Molecular weight*

The average molecular weight of a polymer can be viewed and measured in three different ways as indicated in Table 156.

As these methods of determining the average molecular weight are relatively time-consuming, that of copovidone is now expressed in terms of the K-value, in accordance with the European and U.S. Pharmacopoeia methods for povidone.

The *weight-average* of the molecular weight, $\overline{M}w$ is determined by methods that measure the weights of the individual molecules. The measurement of light scattering has been found to be the most suitable method for polyvinylpyrrolidone [212]. Values determined by this method for copovidone lie between 45 000 and 70 000, depending on the K-value. Recent results do not always agree well with older results, as the apparatus and method used have been improved significantly over the years.

The *number-average* of the molecular weight, $\overline{M}n$ is determined by methods that measure the number of molecules. Values of copovidone recently determined by this method lie between 15000 and 20000.

The *viscosity-average* of the molecular weight, $\overline{M}v$ has attracted greater interest recently, as it can be calculated direct from the intrinsic viscosity [h] (see chapter 2.2.6.2 and 2.3.2.2).

Table 156. Average molecular weights of polymers and their methods of determination

Type of average molecular weight	Symbol	Method of determination
Weight-average	$\overline{Mv}$	Light scattering, ultracentrifuge
Number-average	$\overline{Mn}$	Osmometry, membrane filtration
Viscosity-average	$\overline{Mv}$	Viscosity

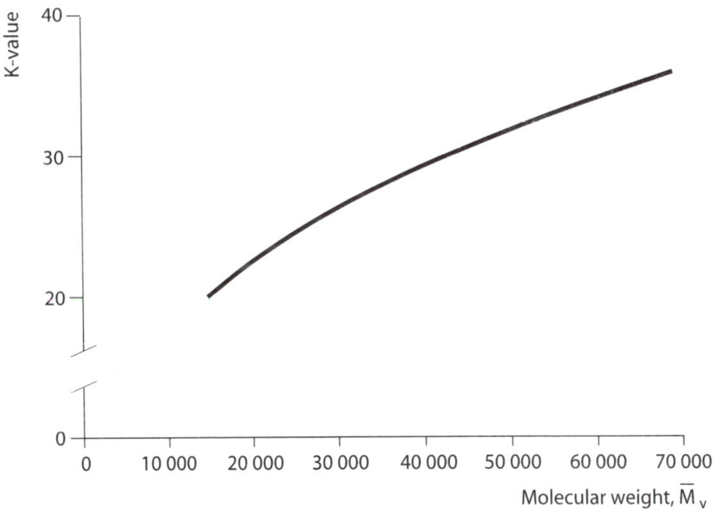

Fig. 92. K-value of as a function of its viscosity average molecular weight, $\overline{Mv}$ [212]

However, it is simpler to calculate $\overline{Mv}$ from the K-value determined by the USP or Ph.Eur. methods, with the following formula [212]:

$$\overline{Mv} = 22.22\ (K + 0.075K^2)^{1.65}$$

The $\overline{Mv}$ values obtained with this equation have been plotted in Fig. 92. They are lower than the $\overline{Mw}$ values, as the equation was developed for the homopolymer, polyvinylpyrrolidone.

4.2.4
Physical properties of the powder

4.2.4.1
Particle size, flowability

When processing auxiliaries such as copovidone in formulations for solid dosage forms, the particle size distribution can be of considerable importance. This particularly applies to the manufacture of tablets. However, it can also be important in solutions, e.g. film-coating solutions for tablets, as the dissolution rate and the dusting properties depend on the proportions of coarse and fine particles respectively.

Copovidone has a relatively low average particle size of about 100 μm and it contains no coarse particles and little fines. Table 157 gives some typical values valid for both commercial products mentioned in Table 151.

The uniform distribution of the particle size (Fig. 93) and also the (partly) spherical particle structure (Fig. 94 and 95) make copovidone free flowing and easy to handle in dry processes.

Table 157. Particle size of copovidone (sieving method, e.g. air jet screen)

Sieve	Value
Smaller than 50 μm	approx. 15 – 20 %
Smaller than 100 μm	approx. 50 – 60 %
Larger than 250 μm	less than 5 %

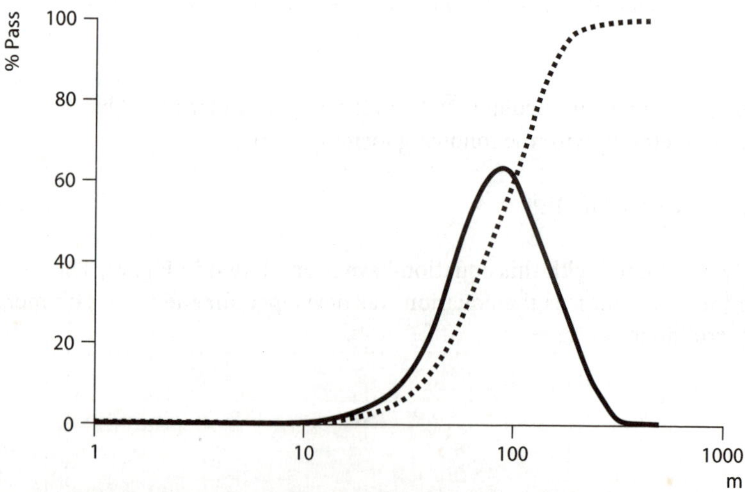

Fig. 93. Typical particle size distribution of copovidone (Plasdone® S-630)

4.2.4.2
Particle structure

Copovidone is a spray dried product like povidone. Therefore the structure of the particles corresponds to this technology. Typical for copovidone are the deformed or partly broken holow spherical particles. This irregular structure is one of the important reasons for the excellent dry binding properties of copovidone in the direct compression technology of tablets. Figures. 94 and 95 illustrate this structure of the two commercial products in the market by means of scanning electron micrographs.

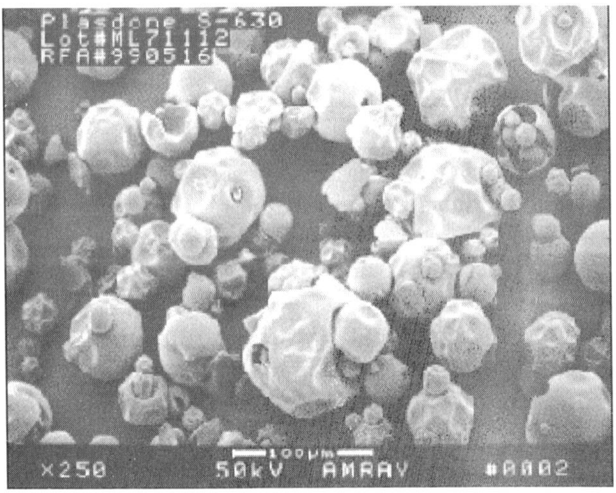

Fig. 94. Electron micrograph of Plasdone® S-630

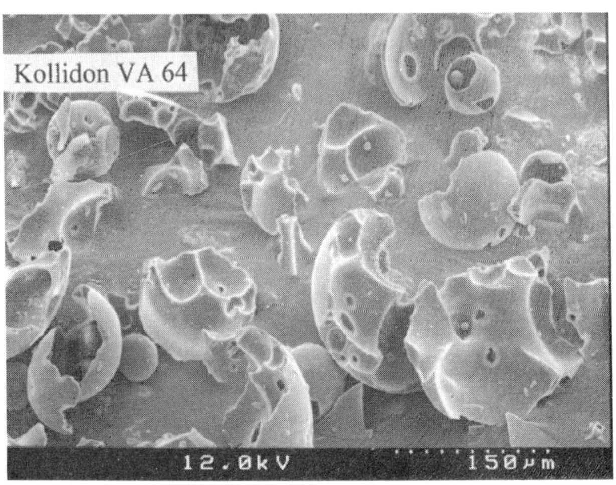

Fig. 95. Electron micrograph of Kollidon® VA 64

Table 158. Bulk and tap density of the commercial copovidone products

	Kollidon® VA 64	Plasdone® S-630
Bulk density	about 0.26 g/ml	about 0.23 g/ml
Tap density	about 0.39 g/ml	about 0.35 g/ml

4.2.4.3
Bulk density, tap density

The bulk density of copovidone is relatively low and does not increase very much with movement. The following typical values can be given (Table 158).

4.2.4.4
Hygroscopicity

The importance of the hygroscopicity of an excipient depends on the application. When it is used as a binder and granulating aid in tablets, a certain degree of hygroscopicity is useful, while in film coatings, it is a nuisance. Overall, copovidone absorbs about 3 times less water than povidone at a given relative humidity, as can be seen from Fig. 96.

As the amount of water absorbed from the air is particularly important in film coating, this was determined with cast copovidone films that contained 2.5% glyc-

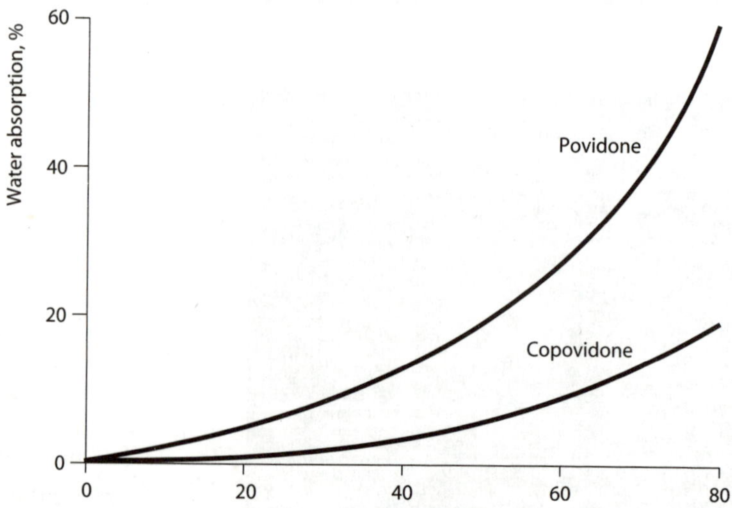

Fig. 96. Hygroscopicity of copovidone and povidone for comparison, after 7 days at 25°C

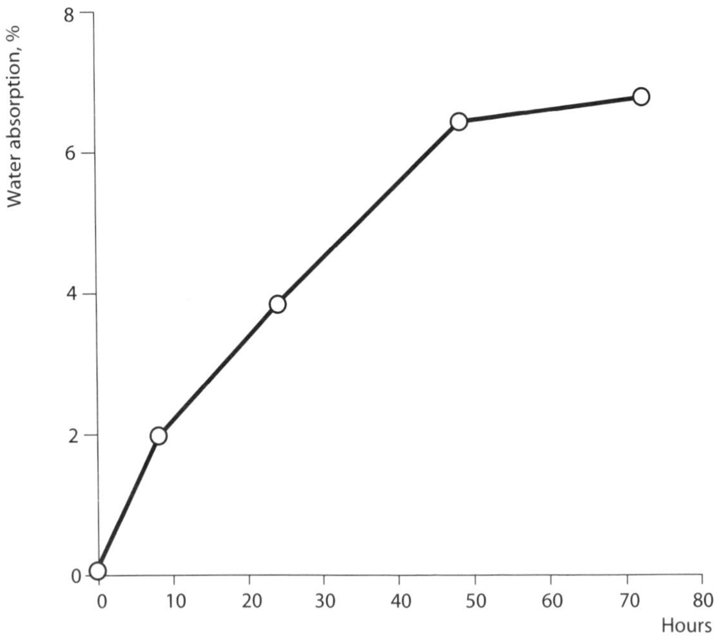

Fig. 97. Water absorption by copovidone films containing 2.5% glycerol, over a period of 72 hours at 25°C and 85% relative humidity

erol as a plasticizer. Figure 97 shows that a film of this type absorbs significantly less water in 80 hours at 85% relative humidity than the powder for which results are given in Fig. 96.

4.2.5 Stability, storage, packaging

Copovidone is very stable when it is stored as the pure product in the sealed, original containers at room temperature (23–25°C). It still meets the specifi-cations given in Section 4.2.1.2 after more than 3 years.

As with povidone, the peroxide content of can increase slowly in the presence of atmospheric oxygen. However, the peroxide level increases much slower than in the case of povidone and it remains much below the required limit of 400 ppm, calculated as H_2O_2.

For the stability of solutions in water the only parameter sensitive during the storage is the colour. If an antioxidant like 0.5% cysteine is added also the colour can be stabilized as can be seen in Table 159.

Table 159. Storage of solutions of 10% copovidone in water at pH 6.4 in the dark during months at 40°C

Parameter	Initial values	Storage under air	Storage under nitrogen	Storage after addition of 0.5% of cysteine
Colour (Ph.Eur.*)	B 6–7	BY 4–5	BY 3–4	BY 6–7
Peroxides	<20 ppm	<20 ppm	<20 ppm	<20 ppm
Saponification value	25	25	25	26
Vinylpyrrolidone	<1 ppm	<1 ppm	<1 ppm	<1 ppm
Clarity**	3,2 FTU	3,2 FTU	3,3 FTU	3,2 FTU

* B = brown, Y = yellow
(The lower the number the stronger the colour intensity)
** FTU = Formazine Turbity Unit

4.3 Analytical methods

4.3.1 Qualitative and quantitative methods of determination

4.3.1.1 *Identification*

Most of the colour and precipitation reactions described in the literature for soluble polyvinylpyrrolidone can be used in the qualitative determination of copovidone (Table 160).

The following further means of distinguishing between copovidone and the homopolymer, povidone are available:

1. Infrared spectrum
   The infrared spectrum provides the clearest identification of copovidone. It differs significantly from that of povidone, as can be seen in Figs. 98 and 99 (arrows indicate differences).
2. Thin-layer chromatography [17]
   Immerse a thin-layer chromatography plate in a 5% solution of paraffin wax in petroleum ether for 5 seconds and dry in the warm. With a n-propanol + 2N ammonia solution (6 + 4 parts by volume) eluent, copovidone gives an Rf value of 0.64–0.75 and povidone an Rf value of 0.59–0.64.
3. Paper chromatography [17]
   On paraffin wax-impregnated filter paper, povidone gives an Rf value of 0.33–0.66 and copovidone an Rf value of 0.72–1.00 with a n-propanol + 2N ammonia solution (6 + 4 parts by volume) eluent.

Table 160. Detection reactions for copovidone and povidone [18]

Reagent	Reaction
10% aqueous barium chloride solution + 1 N hydrochloric acid + 5% aqueous silicotungstic acid solution	White precipitate
10% aqueous barium chloride solution + 1 N hydrochloric acid + 5% aqueous phosphotungstic acid solution	Yellow precipitate
10% potassium dichromate solution + 1 N hydrochloric acid	Orange-yellow precipitate
Saturated aqueous potassium iodide solution + 0.1 N iodine solution	Brown-red precipitate
Dragendorff's reagent + 1 N hydrochloric acid	Brown-red precipitate
Nessler's reagent	Yellowish-white precipitate
Aqueous ammonium-cobalt rhodanide solution + 6 N hydrochloric acid	Blue precipitate

Table 161. Identification reactions for copovidone/copolyvidone in the pharmacopoeias

Reaction	Ph.Eur. 5	JPE 1993
Colour reaction with iodine	+	+
Detection of vinyl acetate part as ethyl acetate	–	+
Detection as the hydroxamic acid with iron(III) chloride	+	–
IR spectrum	+	–

4. Detection as the hydroxamic acid [17]
   Of all the polyvinylpyrrolidone polymers, only copovidone reacts with 3 M hydroxylamine solution to form a hydroxamic acid, which reacts with iron(III) salts to give a violet colour, as described in the Ph.Eur. monograph, "Copovidone".
5. Electrophoresis [17]

The monographs of Ph.Eur. 5 and of JPE 1993 give the identification reactions listed in Table 161. In the Ph. Eur. monograph the infrared spectrum is classified as indendification A and the other reactions are an alternative classified as second identification B.

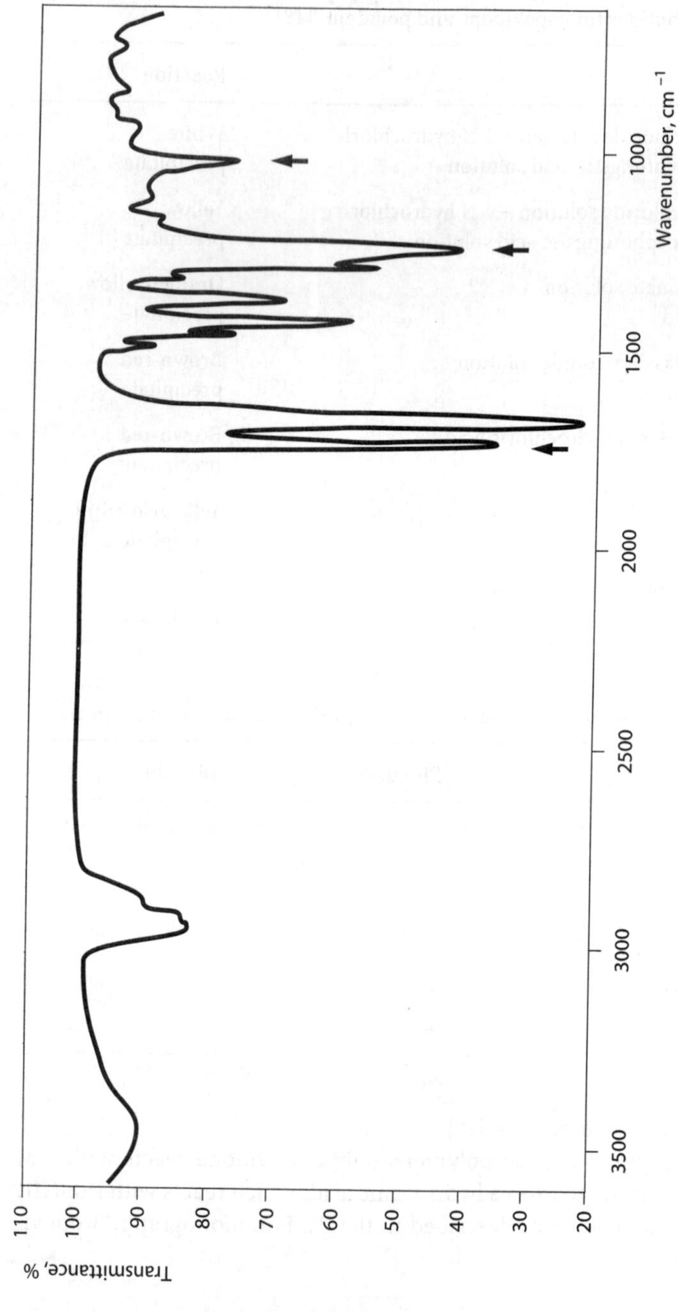

Fig. 98. Infrared spectrum of copovidone recorded in KBr [18]

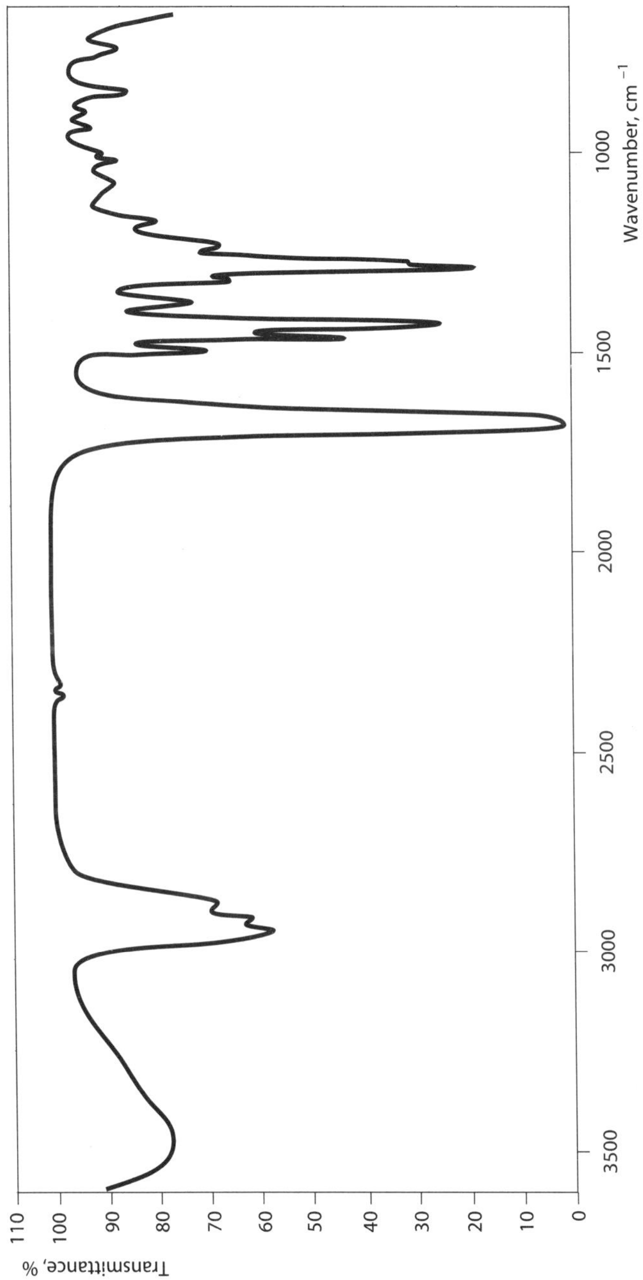

Fig. 99. Infrared spectrum of povidone K 30 in KBr [18]

4.3.1.2
Quantitative methods of determination

The photometric determination of the iodine complex used to determine povidone can also be used for copovidone, though the colour intensity of the iodine complex only reaches its maximum after about 30 min, after which it slowly fades. Thus, it must be measured after 30 min, instead of 10 min, as in the determination of povidone [18].

Mix 50 ml of the sample solution, which must contain less than 50 μg of copovidone/ml with 25 ml of 0.2 M citric acid solution. Mix this with 10 ml of 0.006 N iodine solution (0.81 g of freshly sublimed iodine and 1.44 g of potassium iodide dissolved in 1000 ml of water), and measure the absorbance of this solution against that of a blank solution (50 ml of water + 25 ml of 0.2 M citric acid solution + 10 ml of 0.006 N iodine solution) at 420 nm after exactly 30 min.

A calibration curve must be established to determine the copovidone content from the absorbance (Fig. 100). The absorbance of the iodine complex is slightly less than that of the povidone-iodine complex.

The method for the quantitative determination of copovidone given by the Ph.Eur. monograph measures the nitrogen content (theoretical value 7.1%) by the Kjeldahl method.

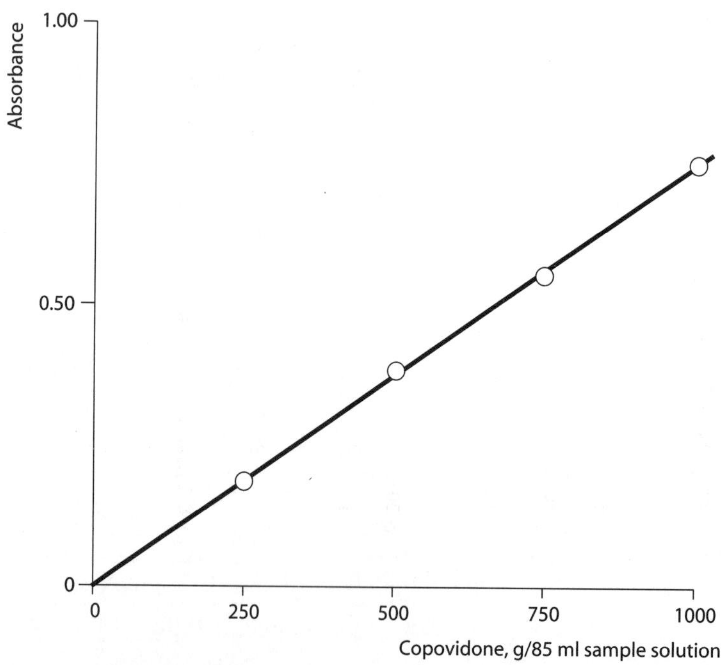

Fig. 100. Calibration curve for the photometric determination of copovidone with iodine [18]

Table 162. Purity test methods for copovidone given in the pharmacopoeias

Acetaldehyde
Monomers (sum of N-vinylpyrrolidone + vinyl acetate)
Hydrazine
Peroxides
Nitrogen
Colour and clarity in solution
Loss on drying
Sulfated ash/residue on ignition
Heavy metals
K-value
2-Pyrrolidone
Polymerized vinyl acetate (Saponification value)
Residual solvents
Microbial status

4.3.2 Methods for the determination of purity

4.3.2.1 *Pharmacopoeia methods*

Methods for determining the purity of copovidone are described in the corresponding monograph of Ph.Eur. The parameters measured are those given in Table 162.

Some of the pharmacopoeia methods are not always entirely relevant. This applies particularly to the titration test for the N-vinylpyrrolidone and vinyl acetate monomers, as the method is not very specific and relatively inaccurate and therefore no longer do justice to the purity of copovidone.

For this reason, alternative methods are described in the sections 2.3.3.2 and 4.3.2.2.

4.3.2.2 *HPLC method for the determination of N-vinylpyrrolidone and vinyl acetate in copovidone*

As copovidone almost always contains levels of N-vinylpyrrolidone and vinyl acetate that are much lower than the detection limits of pharmacopoeia titration methods, it is recommended to use a more sensitive method such as high performance liquid chromatography (HPLC).

The following HPLC method was taken from the Ph. Eur. monograph "Povidone" (Impurity A) and adapted to copovidone. It is an alternative to the HPLC method described in section 2.3.3.2 and has a detection limit of 1 ppm of N-vinylpyrrolidone and 20 ppm of vinyl acetate.

Principle:
The sample is dissolved and separated by reversed phase chromatography. The interfering polymeric components of the matrix are removed by switching columns. A programmed UV detector operating at 205 nm and 235 nm, calibrated with an external standard, is used to determine the level of monomer.

Sample preparation:
Weigh approx. 100–200 mg of copovidone accurate to 0.01 mg, into a 25-ml volumetric flask, dissolve in 10 ml of a mixture of water + isopropanol (7 + 3, v/v). Then make up to the mark with the same mixture and shake for 30 minutes. Use aliquots of this solution for the HPLC analysis.

If the N-vinylpyrrolidone content would be greater than 10 ppm, or the vinyl acetate content greater than 200 ppm, the sample weight should be reduced or the solution diluted accordingly.

Preparation of the calibration solutions:
Weigh 40–50 mg of N-vinylpyrrolidone and vinyl acetate, accurate to 0.01 mg, into separate 50-ml volumetric flasks and dissolve in about 20 ml of eluent. Then make up to the mark with eluent.

Prepare a series of dilutions from these stock solutions to cover the expected ranges of N-vinylpyrrolidone and vinyl acetate content in the sample.

Column switching:
The analysis is started with the guard column and separation column in series. After 1-2 minutes, the valves, controlled by the detector programme, switch over such that the eluent flows past the guard column, direct to the separation column.

Table 163. Chromatographic conditions

Guard column:	25 x 4 mm cartridge packed with LiChrospher®60 RP select B, 5 µm (Merck)
Separation column:	250 x 4 mm steel column packed with LiChrospher 60 RP select B, 5 µm (Merck)
Eluent (mobile phase):	Water/acetonitrile 92 + 8 (% w/w)
Flow rate:	1.0–1.2 ml/min
Sample volume:	30 µl (vinyl acetate) and 20 µl (vinylpyrrolidone)
Pressure:	About 200 bar
Column temperature:	40 °C
Retention time:	9–11 min (vinyl acetate) and 12-14 min (vinylpyrrolidone)
Detection:	205 nm (vinyl acetate), 235 nm (N-vinylpyrrolidone)

The columns are switched when the components to be determined, but not the interfering matrix, have already reached the separation column. Simultaneously, the guard column is washed out in the reverse direction by a second pump to remove the unwanted matrix components.

After 18–20 minutes, the valves are reset to the starting position for the next analysis.

Figure 103 shows typical chromatograms obtained with these conditions.

Calculation

Calibration factor:

$$F = \frac{A_{St}}{W_{St}}$$

A_{St} = calibration substance peak area [mV s]
W_{St} = weight of calibration substance per 100 ml [mg/100 ml]

Samples:
The content of the sample is calculated with the aid of an external standard:

$$\text{ppm N-vinylpyrrolidone or vinyl acetate} = \frac{A}{F\,W_{Sa}}\ 10^6$$

A = peak area of the sample [mV s]
W_{Sa} = sample weight [mg/100 ml]

Validation

Linearity:
The calibration curves were plotted from 5-7 points covering a broad concentration range to check their linearity. Figures. 101 and 102 show the calibration curves obtained.

Reproducibility:
The N-vinylpyrrolidone and vinyl acetate contents of a copovidone sample were determined 6 times. The values found and the average are given in Table 164.

Recovery rate:
To a sample of one batch of copovidone five different amounts of vinyl acetate and three different amounts of vinylpyrrolidone were added (Tables 165 and 166, Fig. 103).

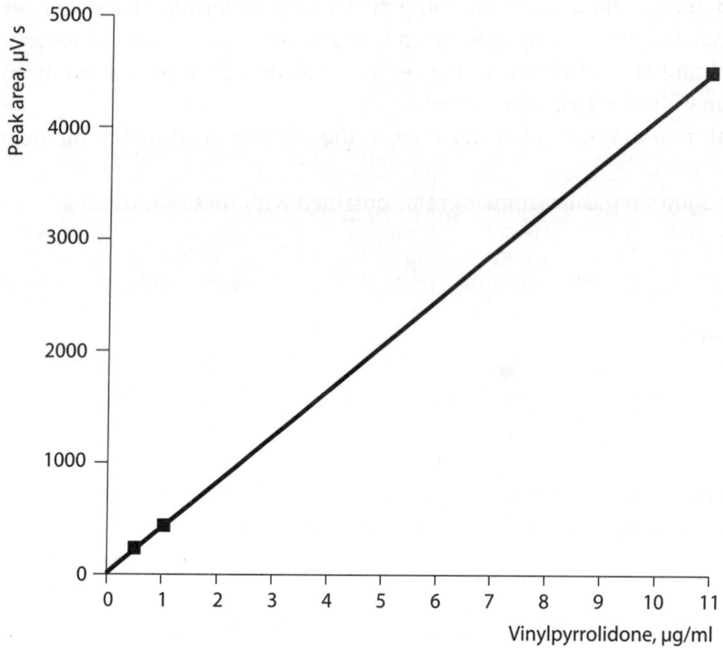

Fig. 101. Calibration curve for the HPLC determinaton of vinylpyrrolidone in copovidone

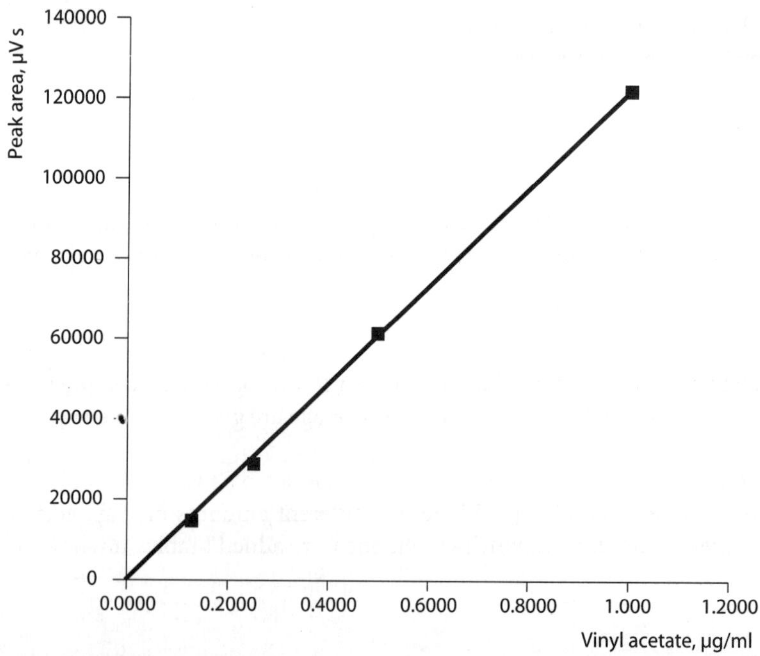

Fig. 102. Calibration curve for the HPLC determinaton of vinyl acetate in copovidone

Table 164. Repeated determination of the monomers in one sample of Kollidon® VA64

Determination No.	Content of vinyl acetate, [mg/kg]	N-vinylpyrrolidone, [mg/kg]
1	15	3
2	19	2
3	18	3
4	19	3
5	18	4
Average	18	3

Table 165. Recovery rate of vinyl acetate

Initial value [mg/kg]	Added vinyl acetate [mg/kg]	Theoretical content [mg/kg]	Found content [mg/kg]	Recovery rate [%]
17.2	13.3	30.5	27.5	77.4
17.2	27.1	44.3	39.9	83.8
17.2	66.3	83.5	79.4	93.8
17.2	100.2	117.4	110.3	92.9
17.2	132.7	1149.9	142.1	94.1

Table 166. Recovery rate of vinylpyrrolidone

Initial value [mg/kg]	Added vinylpyrrolidone [mg/kg]	Theoretical content [mg/kg]	Found content [mg/kg]	Recovery rate [%]
3	5.8	8.8	8.0	86
3	10.0	13.0	12.2	92
3	14.6	17.6	16.3	91

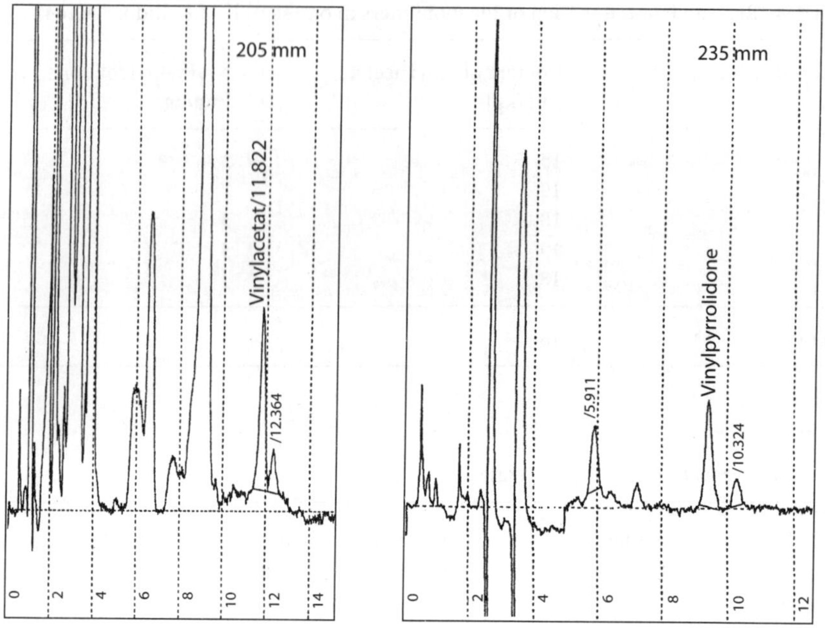

Fig. 103. Typical HPLC chromatograms of copovidone

4.3.2.3
GC Determination of (hydroxy-methyl)-butylpyrrolidone (= "2-propanol-vinyl-pyrrolidone adduct") in copovidone

Because copovidone usually is polymerized in 2-propanol very small amounts of the radical adduct of 2-propanol to the monomer N-vinylpyrrolidone shown in Fig. 32 can be formed (see Section 2.3.3.7).

The gaschromatographic method for the determination of HMBP in copovidone is exactly the same method as described in Section 2.3.3.7 for the low-molecular povidones .

Validation: Recovery in copovidone
In addition to the validation tests reported in Section 2.3.3.7 the recovery rate was determined using copovidone. The content of the 2-propanol-vinyl-pyrrolidone adduct (HMBP) was determined twice on one batch before and after addition of different amounts of HMBP. Table 167 shows the results.

Table 167. Recovery of HMBP in copovidone

	Initial value [mg/kg]	Added amount [mg/kg]	Theoretical content [mg/kg]	Found content [mg/kg]	Recovery rate [%]
Kollidon® VA64 (batch 349)	94	101	195	170	87
Kollidon® VA64 (batch 349)	94	333	427	367	86

4.3.2.4
Determination of acetic acid

The content of the residual solvent acetic acid in copovidone is determined by the following HPLC method using acetic acid as external standard.

Sample solution:
Dissolve 200 mg of the sample in 3.0 ml of methanol, add 20 ml of water and 2 ml of water adjusted with phosphoric acid to pH 0.8 and shake for some seconds. Filtrate immediately about 2 ml of the obtained suspension through a 0.45 µm filter.

Calibration factor and linearity:
The linearity of the calibration of acetic acid was determined in the range of 2.8–22.1 mg/l. Figure 104 shows the result.

The calibration factor is calculated by the following formula:

$$c = \frac{A_r}{W_r}\left[\frac{mV \cdot s}{mg/100ml}\right]$$

Table 168. Chromatographic conditions:

Precolumn:	Lichrospher 100 RP 18, 5 µm, 25 mm x 4 mm(Merck)
Main column:	Lichrospher 100 RP 18, 5 µm, 250 mm x 4 mm (Merck)
Column temperatures:	30 °C
Mobile phase:	Water, adjusted with phosphoric acid to pH 2.4
Flow rate:	0.9 ml/min
Pressure:	about 150 bar
Injection volume:	10 µl
Detection wavelength:	205 nm
Retention time of acetic acid:	about 4.3 min

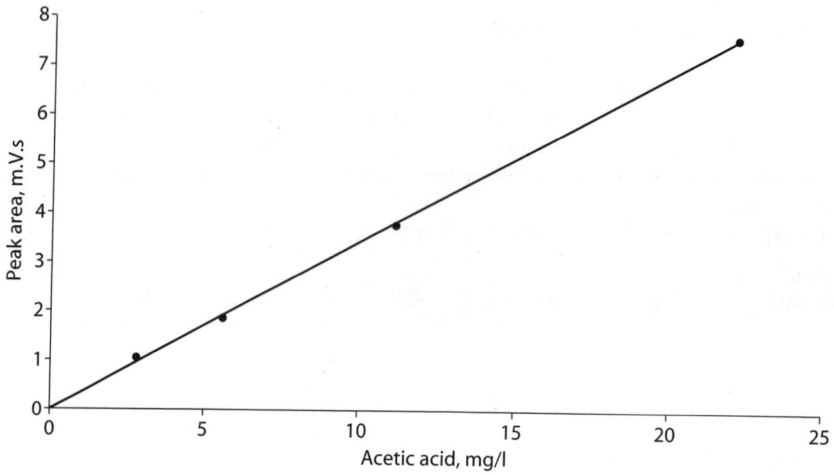

Fig. 104. Calibration curve of acetic acid

A_r = Area of the peak of active acid reference sustance [mV · s]
W_r = Weight of acetic acid reference substance [mg/100 ml]

Calculation of the content of acetic acid in the sample

$$\text{Acetic acid (\%)} = \frac{A_s \times 100}{C \times W_S}$$

As = Area of the acetic acid peak of the sample solution [mV· s]
C = Calipraction factor
W_s = Sample weight [mg/100 ml]
A typical chromatogram obtained with this method is shown in Fig. 105.

Reproducibility:
The content of acetic acid was determined 5 times in a sample and the following results were obtained (Table 169).

Recovery rate:
See Table 170.

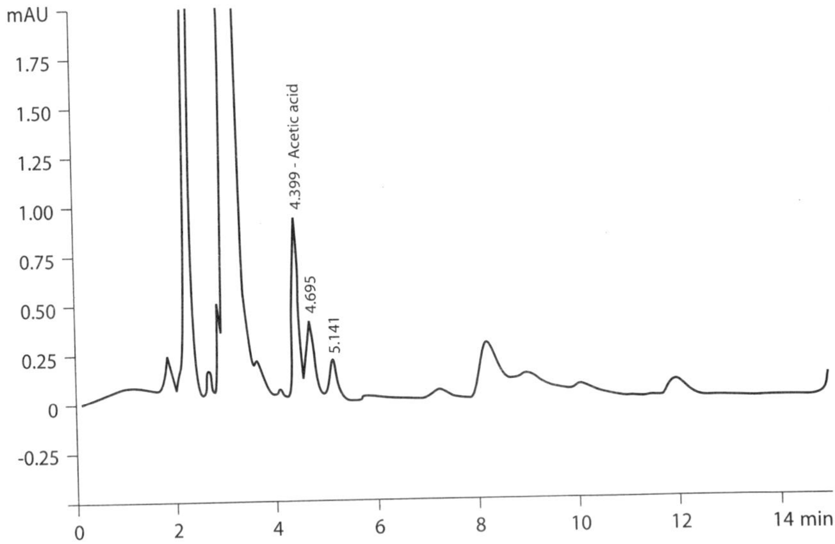

Fig. 105. Typical chromatogram of acetic acid in a sample

Table 169. Reproducibility of the determination of acetic acid in a sample

Measurement	Acetic acid
1	0.274
2	0.262
3	0.257
4	0.251
5	0.255
Average	0.260

Table 170. Recovery of added acetic acid in a sample

Added acetic acid, ppm	Theoretical content of acetic acid, %	Found acetic acid, %	Recovery rate, %
0	0.2600	0.260	–
103	0.2703	0.271	100.3
153	0.2753	0.274	99.5
204	0.2804	0.278	99.1

4.3.3
Determination of copovidone in preparations

4.3.3.1
Qualitative determination

The detection reactions for copovidone given in Section 4.3.1.1 can be used to detect this copolymer in most pharmaceutical preparations. Should these provide no clear results, the separation scheme shown in Fig. 106 can be used to detect copovidone in solid dosage forms, e.g. tablets, granules, capsules and coated tablets.

The detection and differentiation of povidone and copovidone obtained in Fraction A I in Fig. 106 is best carried out by thin layer chromatography on silica gel or paper. A suitable eluent is a mixture of 6 parts n-propanol and 4 parts 2N ammonia solution by volume, with which copovidone gives a higher Rf value than povidone (see Section 4.3.1.1).

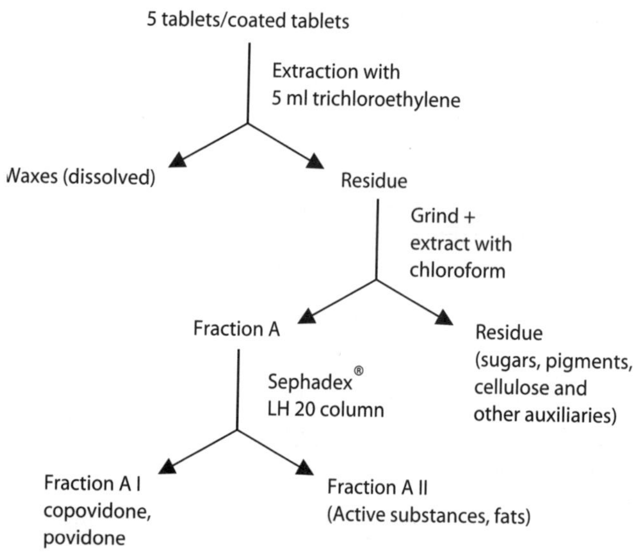

Fig. 106. Separation scheme for the detection of copovidone in solid dosage forms [17]

Sephadex® is a registered trademark of Amersham Biosciences AB, Uppsala, Sweden

Table 171. Determination of copovidone as the iodine complex in the presence of active substances and auxiliaries [18]

	μg of copovidone, recovered in the presence of 20 times the quantity of:			
Copovidone added, μg	Thiamine hydrochloride	Caffeine	Acetphene-tidine	Lactose
50	49	48	49	48
100	102	100	102	96
200	203	201	203	198

4.3.3.2
Quantitative determination in preparations

The most versatile method for quantitatively determining copovidone is probably the photometric measurement of the iodine complex described in Section 4.3.1.2. It has been successfully tested on samples that also contained a series of auxiliaries and active substances, to verify its suitability for preparations.

In these tests, aqueous solutions containing 50, 100 and 200 μg of copovidone and 20 times the quantity of the tablet ingredients listed in Table 171 were prepared, and their copovidone content determined.

4.4
Applications of copovidone

4.4.1
General notes

The vinylpyrrolidone-vinyl acetate copolymer has been used by the pharmaceutical industry in Europe for decades [101, 114, 231, 409]. Up to about 1975, it was sold in this sector under tradenames, which are now used exclusively for the technical/cosmetic grade of this copolymer. This is why many older publications often mention one of these tradenames (e.g. Luviskol®* VA64) for use in pharmaceutical products.

The applications of copovidone rely mainly on its good binding and film-forming properties, its affinity to hydrophilic and hydrophobic surfaces and its relatively low hygroscopicity. Because of these properties, it is mainly used as a processing aid in the production of granules and tablets, as a binder in direct compression, in film coatings on tablets, as a protective layer and subcoat for tablet cores and as a film-forming agent in sprays.

* Luviskol® is a registered trademark of of BASF AG, Ludwigshafen, Germany

The advantage over povidone in solid dosage forms lies mainly in its lower hygroscopicity and higher plasticity (see Sections 4.2.4.4 and 4.4.2.4). Copovidone is seldom used in liquid dosage forms, apart from sprays.

4.4.2
Binder for tablets, granulates and hard gelatin capsules

4.4.2.1
General notes

The main area of application of copovidone is as a binder in tablets and granules (including granules for hard gelatin capsules), regardless of whether they are made by wet or dry granulation or by direct compression (see Fig. 36 in Section 2.4.2.1), as it is equally effective in all three cases. It can also be used in extrusion [465] or in cocrystallization [463].

The usual concentration in which copovidone is used as a binder in tablets and granules lies between 2% and 5%. This range is similar to that of povidone K 30 in tablets.

4.4.2.2
Manufacture of tablets and pellets by wet granulation

Granulation is still the most frequently used method of preparing a tabletting mixture. There are at least four different variations of the procedure (Table 172).

Water is nowadays the most commonly used solvent. Sometimes, if water cannot be used, as with effervescent tablets, active ingredients that are prone to hydrolysis etc., ethanol or isopropanol are used as solvents, though fluidized bed granulation is preferred.

There are a number of factors that dictate which of the methods in Table 172 must be used. With some formulations, Method 1 gives tablets with a shorter disintegration time and quicker release of the active substance than Method 2 [314]. In many cases, Method 1 gives somewhat harder tablets than Method 2. Method 3 in Table 172 is useful if Method 1 cannot be used, as when the tabletting mixture

Table 172. Methods of wet granulation with a binder

1. Granulation of the active substance (+ filler) with a binder solution.
2. Granulation of the active substance (+ filler)-binder mixture with the pure solvent.
3. Granulation of a mixture of the active substance (+ filler) and a portion of the binder with a solution of the remaining binder.
4. Granulation of the active substance (+ filler) with the solution of a portion of the binder followed by dry addition of the remaining binder to the finished granulate.

lacks the capacity for the quantity of liquid required for the total amount of binder. If the disintegration time of a tablet presents a problem, it is worth trying Method 4, mixing in about a third of the binder together with lubricant and, last of all, the disintegrant.

Methods 2 and 3 have proved best for active substances of high solubility, as the quantity of liquid can be kept small to avoid clogging the granulating screens.

As a typical example of Method 1 of Table 172. Figure 107 shows that there are no significant differences in the compression diagrams for povidone K 25, povidone K 30 and copovidone for lactose placebo tablets containing 3% of each binder. The results are only valid for the wet granulation technology because the use as dry binder gives a higher hardness in the case of copovidone than of other binders (see Fig. 111 and Table 174).

In other cases of wet granulation according to Method 1 of Tablet 172 it was also not possible to measure any major differences in the hardness of corn starch-lactose tablets granulated with copovidone and povidone K 30, over the usual range of binder proportions. However, the hardness of tablets made with hydroxypropyl cellulose (Type L) was much lower. Similar results were obtained with calcium phosphate tablets.

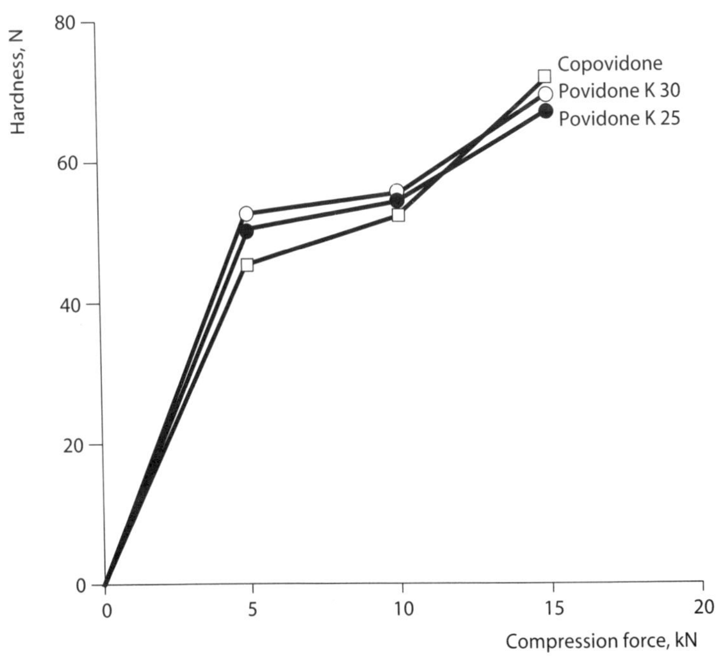

Fig. 107. Effect of the compression force on the hardness of lactose tablets containing 3 % copovidone compared with tablets containing 3% povidone K 25 or povidone K 30 (only valid for wet granulation, Method 1)

As can be seen from Fig. 108 copovidone has the advantage over povidone K 30 in the solvent granulation technology (Method 2 of Table 172) that small quantities of water used as granulation liquid give a higher tablet hardness.

The capacity of the powder mixture to bind liquid is one of the parameters that can be used to determine the quantity of binder solution required in wet granulation. Every powder mixture to be granulated has a different adsorption capacity for the solvent or the copovidone solutions, which most effectively minimizes the proportion of fines [483].

With all four of the granulating methods in Table 172, copovidone usually gives hard tablets or pellets of low friability. Since it is soluble, the drug normally dissolves rapidly, whether in gastric or intestinal juice [132, 644] and frequently relatively independently of the compression force, as can be seen in Fig. 109. Like in the case of povidone K 30 it can be expected that copovidone enhances the dissolution of many drugs as shown with griseofulvin [528].

An important property of copovidone, in its use as a binder for tablets, is its plasticity [68c], a property that povidone does not possess (see Fig. 110). This property gives granules and mixtures that are less susceptible to capping during compression, and tablets that are less brittle. The tablets also have less tendency to stick to the punches when tabletting machines are operated under humid conditions.

Two formulations, for ampicillin and cimetidine tablets, that have been developed on a laboratory scale, are given in Table 173 as examples for the use of copovidone in the binder solution granulation. It is also highly suitable for producing preparations such as multivitamin granules [368 c].

Copovidone is also an excellent binder for the production of pellets. Typical examples are spheronized pellets of propranolol and verapamil [615] and pellets of theophylline [479].

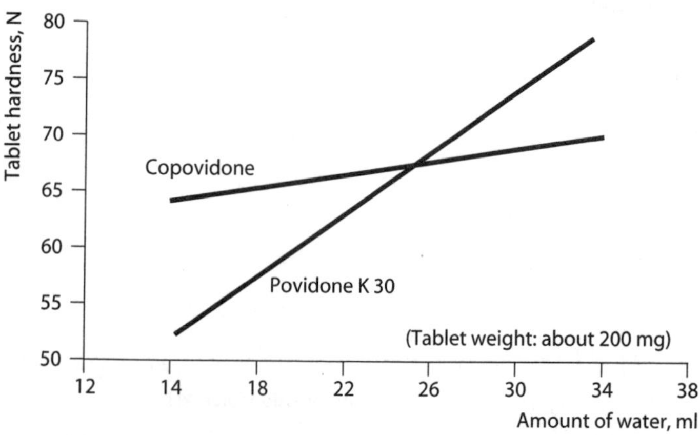

Fig. 108. Influence of the amount of water as granulation liquid on the tablet hardness (Solvent granulation of tablets of 100 mg of aminophylline [615])

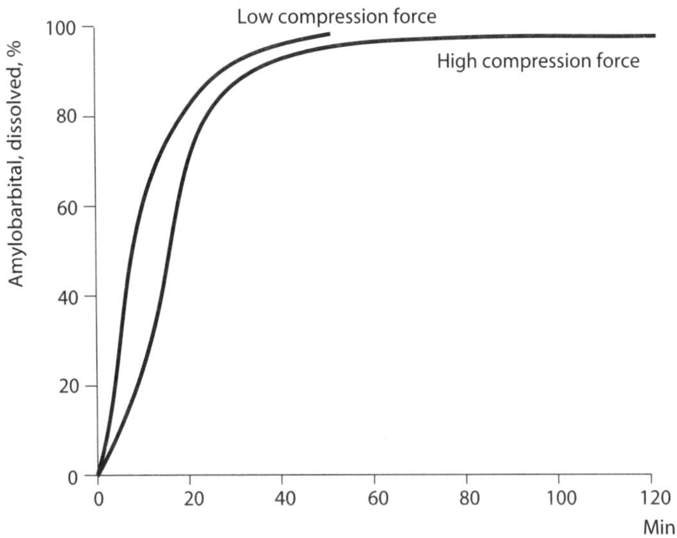

Fig. 109. Influence of the compression force on the dissolution of amylobarbital from tablets granulated with copovidone [132]

Table 173. Ampicillin tablets (500 mg) and cimetidine tablets (400 mg) [615]

1. Formulations

I	Ampicillin trihydrate	500 g	–
	Cimetidine	–	400 g
	Corn starch	242 g	170 g
II	Copovidone	25 g	20 g
	2-Propanol or water	q. s.	q. s.
III	Crospovidone	15 g	–
	Magnesium stearate	10 g	3 g
	Aerosil® 200	8 g	–

Granulate mixture I with solution II, dry and sieve, mix with III and press into tablets with a low pressure.

Tablets obtained on a laboratory scale with a rotary tabletting machine had the following properties:

2. Tablet properties

Weight		798 mg	601 mg
Hardness		170 N	91 N
Disintegration in gastric juice		5 min	4 min
Friability		0.35%	0.5%
Dissolution (USP)	20 min	Not	91%
	30 min	tested	100%

4.4.2.3
Manufacture of tabletting mixtures by roller compaction

Dry granulation is less widely used than wet granulation as a method for preparing tabletting mixtures. The best-known dry granulation technique is the roller compaction. It is the method of choice whenever wet granulation cannot be used for reasons of stability and the physical properties of the drug do not allow direct compression. Copovidone is also very suitable as a binder in this type of granulation [637, 653].

4.4.2.4
Direct compression

Direct compression is now becoming ever more widely used, even though most drugs cannot readily be directly compressed in the desired concentrations. For good tabletting properties, a drug must fulfil a number of physical requirements. It must be free-flowing, it must not be prone to electrostatic charging, its crystals must not be too brittle and its compression characteristics must result in tablets of adequate hardness.

Although most drug substances do not fulfil these criteria, they can be directly compressed with copovidone [68c, 213, 458, 459, 464, 615]. It could be considered as the best dry binder of all substances usually applied in drugs for this purpose. The main reasons of the excellent dry binder properties are the plasticity shown in Fig. 110, the lower glass transition temperature (see Section 4.4.3.1) and the irregular structure of its particles (see Figs. 94 and 95 in Section 4.2.4.2).

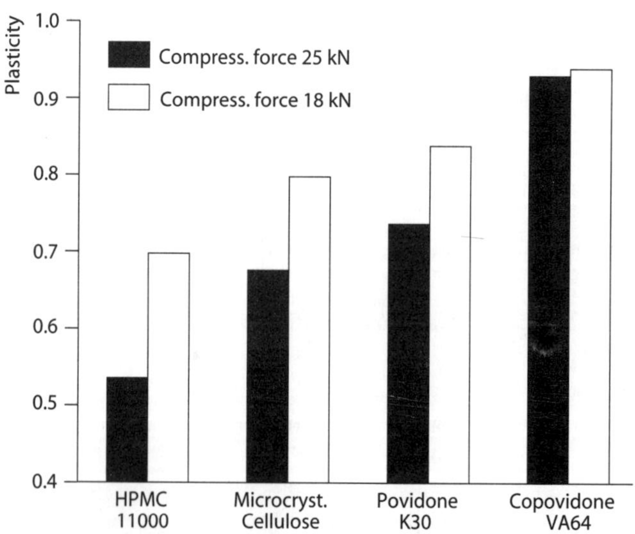

Fig. 110. Plasticity of different dry binders mixed with 0.5% of magnesium stearate in tablets (Plasticity = plastic energy/total energy)

The hardness, friability, porosity and disintegration time of lactose and starch placebo tablets made with copovidone were directly related to the compression force used [458].

Excellent direct compression systems can be formulated with a combination of about 5% copovidone with fillers such as lactose, microcrystalline cellulose, sorbitol or mannitol, and, if required, a disintegrant, a flow improver and/or a lubricant. These have been successfully tested in combination with more than 30 drugs [213, 464, 615].

These combinations are also very good for single-vitamin or multivitamin tablets [368e]. In tablets with several vitamins, they provide superior chemical stability, by avoiding the need for wet granulation, with equally good physical properties [615].

It is normally difficult to produce tablets with ascorbic acid by direct compression, but as is shown in Table 174, they can be produced much more readily using copovidone. When this dry binder is added, the hardness of the tablets increases and the friability decreases much more than after the addition of povidone K 30 or hydroxypropylmethylcellulose (HPMC) which had no effect on the hardness in this formulation. Similar results were shown in Fig. 111 for acetaminophen tablets.

The combination of copovidone with sucrose and microcrystalline cellulose is mentioned for vitamin C chewable tablets in the commentary to the German Standard Generic Formulations as show in Table 175 [460].

Table 176 shows how it was possible to considerably improve the tabletting properties of an antiacid tablet containing alginic acid, magnesium trisilicate, aluminium hydroxide and sodium hydrogen carbonate as the active principles by the addition of copovidone. The hardness was doubled and the friability reduced by half.

Table 174. Dry binding effect of different dry binders in ascorbic acid tablets

Formulations	Without binder	Copovidone	Povidone K 30	HPMC 11 000
Ascorbic acid	200 g	200 g	200 g	200 g
Ludipress®	256 g	256 g	256 g	256 g
Copovidone	–	25 g	–	–
Povidone K 30	–	–	25 g	–
HPMC 11 000	–	–	–	25 g
Crospovidone	15 g	15 g	15 g	15 g
Aerosil® 200	1.2 g	1.2 g	1.2 g	1.2 g
Magnesium stearate	2.5 g	2.5 g	2.5 g	2.5 g
Tablet properties (lab scale, rotary press):				
Hardness	**56 N**	**73 N**	**59 N**	**57 N**
Friability	**3.2%**	**0.4%**	**1.1%**	**0.9%**
Dissolution (30 min)	>90%	>90%	>90%	>90%

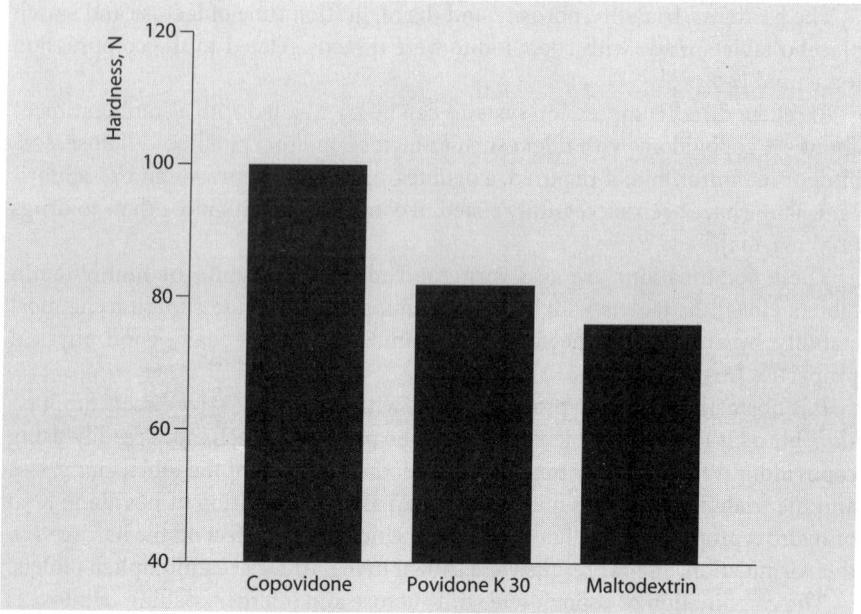

Fig. 111. Influence of the type of dry binder on the hardness of acetaminophen tablets 500 mg obtained by direct compression (3.5% dry binder, tablet weight 700 mg, compression force 25 kN)

Table 175. Ascorbic acid chewable tablets (100 mg)

Formulation (direct compression) [460]

Ascorbic acid, powder	42.2%
Sucrose, ground	13.0%
Sucrose, crystalline	8.0%
Microcrystalline cellulose	28.3%
Copovidone	2.4%
Polyethylene glycol 6000, powder	2.0%
Orange flavour + strawberry flavour (2 + 1)	1.2%
Cyclamate sodium	2.4%
Saccharine sodium	0.1%
Silicagel	0.2%

Tablet properties

Tablets pressed on a rotary tabletting press in the BASF laboratories had the following properties:

Weight	250 mg
Diameter	8 mm
Hardness	157 N
Disintegration in water	15 min
Friability	less than 0.1%

Table 176. Improvement in the properties of antiacid tablets with the addition of copovidone

Formulation (direct compression)		
Alginic acid	500 g	500 g
Magnesium trisilicate	25 g	25 g
Aluminium hydroxide dried gel	100 g	100 g
Sodium bicarbonate	170 g	170 g
Sorbitol, cryst.	160 g	160 g
Sucrose, cryst.	627 g	627 g
Ludipress®	900 g	900 g
Magnesium stearate	50 g	50 g
Vanillin	5 g	5 g
Copovidone	–	70 g

Tablets produced in the laboratory on a rotary tabletting machine with a compression force of 30 kN had the following properties:

Weight	2504 mg	2550 mg
Diameter	20 mm	20 mm
Hardness	67 N	120 N
Friability	3.0 %	1.3 %

In direct compression, particular attention must be paid to the moisture in the tabletting mixture, although under normal conditions the usual residual quantities of water in copovidone suffice to provide an adequate binding effect between the particles.

4.4.2.5
Granules, hard gelatin capsules

The binding properties of copovidone described in Sections 4.4.2.1 and 4.4.2.2, that are of advantage in wet granulation, can, of course, also be used in the production of granules as a dosage form or for filling into hard gelatin capsules. The most important functions of copovidone here are to enlarge the size of the granules, to achieve good flow properties and to avoid dusting. This makes the granules easier to handle when they are filled into containers or hard gelatin capsules.

4.4.3
Tablet coatings

4.4.3.1
Film coatings

Copovidone forms soluble films, independently of the pH, regardless of whether it is processed as a solution in water or in organic solvents, or as a powder. It differs from povidone as a film-forming agent in that it is less hygroscopic (see Section 4.2.4.4) and has greater plasticity and elasticity. At the same time the films are also less tacky. The glass transition temperature depends on the moisture content, and at 103°C for dry copovidone, is also below that of dry povidone K 30 (168°C).

Pure isolated films of copovidone were found to have a failure energy of only 1 J/m² at room temperature – a measure of their tack. The failure energy of povidone K 30 films was 45 J/m2. As copovidone usually absorbs too much water, it can seldom be used as the sole film-forming agent in a formulation. It is therefore recommended to combine it with less hygroscopic substances such as cellulose derivatives [101, 117], shellac, polyvinyl alcohol, polyethylene glycol (e.g. macrogol 6000) or sucrose. Plasticizers such as triethyl citrate, triacetin or phthalates are not normally required. The typical formulations given in Tables 177 to 178 were tested in the laboratory on tablet cores of 9 mm diameter weighing 200 mg.

The properties of coatings can be significantly improved with copovidone, particularly when it is combined with cellulose derivatives [580, 620]. In the case of the tablet film coating using HPMC 2910 the viscosity of the spray suspension containing 12% of polymer can be decreased from about 700 mPa · s to 250 mPa.s if 60% of the HPMC polymer is sustituted [615]. Since the viscosity of 250 mPa.s

Table 177. Film coating with HPMC (Accela Cota 240″)

I.	Copovidone	53 g
	Macrogol 6000	12 g
	HPMC 2910 (6 mPa · s)	79 g
	Water	732 g
II.	Titanium dioxide	36 g
	Iron oxide red	18 g
	Talc	54 g
	Water	216 g

Mix solution I with suspension II, pass through a disc mill and spray with 2 bar onto 5 kg of cores. The quantity of film former applied is about 3 mg/cm².

Inlet/outlet air temperature	60°C/40°C
Spraying rate	50 g/min
Spraying time (continuously)	34 min
Drying after spraying	5 min at 60°C

Table 178. Sugar-film coating (Accela Cota 24″)

Sucrose	40 g
Copovidone	10 g
Macrogol 4000	8 g
Colour lake or iron oxide pigment	3 g
Titanium dioxide	6 g
Talc	10 g
Water	ad 240 g

1200 g of this suspension was sprayed continuously with the pressure of 2 bar onto 5 kg of tablet cores that contained 5% crospovidone as a disintegrant, under the following conditions:

Coating pan speed	15 rpm
Spraying nozzle	0.8 mm
Inlet/outlet air temperature	45°C/36°C
Spraying time	50 min
Quantity applied	Approx. 4 mg of film-forming agents/cm^2

is considered as the usual limit for spraying of a coating suspension such substitution permits to apply this high polymer concentration and therefore to economize the spraying procedure.

It can be used together with shellac, which is a natural product and therefore subject to variations in quality, to obtain films with more consistent properties.

A more recent and most interesting variation on the theme of film coatings with copovidone is its combination with sucrose to produce "sugar-film coated" tablets. Here, copovidone performs all the functions listed in Table 84, mainly film formation and inhibition of crystallization, to give a time and material-saving coating. Table 178 gives a formulation for such a coating. Film coated tablets with even films were obtained after only 50 min.

As an alternative to processing copovidone in solutions in water and/or organic solvents, it can be applied to the tablet cores in powder form at 40°C with the aid of a plasticizer such as triacetin to reduce the film-forming temperature [466].

4.4.3.2
Subcoating of tablet cores as a barrier to water

As tablets are nowadays coated mostly with aqueous solutions or dispersions, it has become increasingly necessary to provide the tablet cores with a barrier layer prior to sugar or film-coating. This is mainly to protect water-sensitive drugs against hydrolysis and chemical interactions, e.g. between different vitamins, etc. and to prevent the swelling of high-performance tablet disintegrants that are very sensitive even to small quantities of water. Table 89 in Section 2.4.4.3 shows that copovidone is also capable of hydrophilizing the tablet core surface, improving its adhesion properties and reducing dust formation [101].

The subcoating with copovidone is best applied in the same apparatus in which the subsequent sugar or film coating is to be applied. An adequate barrier can be applied with less than 0.5 mg of copovidone/cm2 of the warm tablet cores, using a 10% solution of the copolymer in 2-propanol or ethanol.

4.4.3.3
Traditional sugar coating

Copovidone can be used in the same way as povidone in manual or automized sugar coating, in which it has the advantages of lower hygroscopicity and higher elasticity. Table 84 in Section 2.4.4.1 gives the most important properties and functions of copovidone in sugar coatings.

Sugar coatings are particularly susceptible to cracking when they are applied to large batches of tablet cores that are dried rapidly. As most active substances are hydrophobic, copovidone is useful as an additive to prevent the tablet coating cracking away from the tablet core during manufacture.

Copovidone can certainly be used just as well as povidone K 30 in automatic sugar coating (see Section 2.4.4.1).

4.4.4
Film-forming agent in sprays

Because of its good film-forming properties, its bioadhesion and its good solubility in water, copovidone can also be used as a film-forming agent in water-based sprays for human or veterinary topical administration. Table 179 gives a formulation developed on a laboratory scale for a wound spray containing polidocanol as the active ingredient.

As with film coatings for tablets, a combination of copovidone with a cellulose derivative can also be used for spray solutions, as this both improves the solubility of ethylcellulose and reduces the hygroscopicity of a pure copovidone film.

Table 179. Polidocanol wound spray [615]

Polidocanol	5 g
Macrogol 400	20 g
Copovidone	50 g
Ethylcellulose 20	50 g
Ethyl acetate	675 g
2-Propanol	200 g

Fill the solution into spray cans with the necessary quantity of propellant (e.g. propane/butane).

Table 180. Clotrimazole plaster spray [467]

Clotrimazole	1.0 g
Benzyl alcohol	4.0 g
Isopropyl myristate	6.0 g
Copovidone	12.5 g
2-Propanol	ad 100.0 ml

Fill 6–8 parts of this solution with 2–4 parts of propellant, e.g. propane/butane, into spray cans.

The formulation in Table 180 is an example of an antimycotic film plaster spray containing the drug, clotrimazole. Here, copovidone is used as the sole film-forming agent.

Similar topical formulations containing steroids, antibiotics and antimycotics are described in patents [468, 469]. Nifedipine is an example of a drug that is used in sublingual sprays with copovidone [468].

For the veterinary application copovidone is used as filmformer and bioadhesive in fipronil sprays.

4.4.5 Matrix-forming agent in sustained-release and fast-release dosage forms

4.4.5.1 *Sustained-release preparations*

Once it has been pressed as matrix into tablets or melted, copovidone dissolves more slowly than povidone K 30. This property could be used to control or delay the release of drugs, by embedding them in a hydropholic matrix of copovidone. Table 181 lists a number of drugs, mentioned in the literature, that are used with copovidone in sustained-release preparations.

Copovidone has various functions in this application:

1. As the main component, it provides the actual matrix to which lipophilic or water-insoluble substances such as stearic acid and stearyl alcohol [475–476], cellulose derivatives [476], starch [475] or calcium hydrogen phosphate [474] are added.
2. It forms an insoluble complex with polyacrylic acid, in the same way as povidone, (see Section 2.4.8.8) and thus provides the matrix [411, 473].
3. As the hydrophilic component, copovidone controls the release of the drug when it is added to a lipophilic matrix such as stearyl alcohol or cetyl alcohol [471, 472].

The techniques for manufacturing sustained-release preparations with copovidone can vary widely. The simplest form of processing is direct compression

Table 181. Publications of sustained-release preparations with copovidone as the matrix

Drug	Literature source
Bencyclane fumarate	[473]
Captopril	[411]
Chloropyramine HCl	[411, 473]
Dihydroergotamine methanesulfonate	[471]
Dyphylline	[474]
Imipramine	[473]
Potassium chloride	[471]
Ketoprofen	[472]
Nitroglycerin	[411, 473]
Propaphenone	[476]
Riodipine	[472]
Theophylline	[411, 473, 475–476]
Verapamil	[477]

[474]. Other processes involve fluidized bed granulation [411], melt granulation [471], melt extrusion [475–476] or melt compression [477] and powder extrusion [472].

4.4.5.2
Matrix in fast-release preparations

Copovidone can also be used as a matrix in certain rapid-dissolution dosage forms, depending on the other ingredients used [112, 475]. This should be of particular interest for drugs with relatively poor bioavailability, as copovidone forms complexes with these substances, increasing the dissolution rate in much the same manner as does povidone (see Section 2.4.3).

Drugs whose dissolution rate can be increased in this way include carbamazepine [554], pseudoephedrine, diphenhydramine, propaphenon, nicotinic acid, biperiden [475], furosemide [548] and diclofenac.

Further, a copovidone matrix can stabilize certain plant extracts such as valepotriate (valerian extract) [478].

4.4.6
Transdermal and transmucosal systems

Due to its higher plasticity (see Fig. 110), its lower hygroscopicity (see Fig. 96) and its bioadhesion the film former copovidone can be more suitable than povidone for transdermal or transmucosal systems. There is also described a crystallization inhibitory effect of in transdermal/transmucosal systems of dihydroergotamine, melatonine, betamethasone and fusafungine [58, 590]. The bioadhesion of copovidone is used for such systems of oestradiol or levonorgestrel [414], and of flurbiprofen [593].

A typical basic formulation of a mucoadhesive buccal tablet is given in Table 182. In this case the adhesive effect of copovidone was much higher than the adhesion of povidone K 30 or povidone K 90.

Table 182. Basic formulations of a mucoadhesive buccal tablet

		No. 1	No. 2
I	Active ingredient (e.g. morphine sulfate).	q. s.	q. s.
	Lactose monohydrate	76 g	76 g
	Carbopol® 934 (Goodrich)	4 g	–
	Carbopol® 980/981 1 +1 (Goodrich)	–	4 g
	Copovidone	19 g	19 g
II	Ethanol 96%	15 g	10 g
Ill	Magnesium stearate	1 g	1 g

Mix intensively the components I, granulate mixture I with ethanol II, pass through a 0.8 mm sieve, dry, sieve again through a 0.5 mm sieve, mix with the component Ill and press with medium compression force to tablets.

Tablet properties (Formulations No. 1 and No. 2)

Diameter	8 mm
Weight	200 mg
Hardness	> 180 N
Disintegration	> 30 min
Friability	< 0.1%

Buccal adhesive strength (in vitro):
One drop of human saliva was given to a glass plate and a tablet was put on this drop. After 7 min the force (N) needed to separate the tablet vertically from the glass plate was measured:
Formulation No. 1: about 7 N
Formulation No. 2: about 3 N

5 Registration and toxicological data

5.1
Registration

5.1.1
Pharmaceutical products

5.1.1.1
General

An auxiliary such as povidone, crospovidone or copovidone cannot be registered as such by the authorities for use in pharmaceutical products. In Europe, Japan or America, it is always only possible to register a finished drug. There is no general positive or negative list of auxiliaries used in pharmaceuticals. It is only possible to state in which countries pharmaceuticals that contain povidone, copovidone and/or crospovidone are registered.

5.1.1.2
Pharmacopoeias

In practice, a pharmaceutical preparation that contains povidone, copovidone and/or crospovidone can only be registered if these auxiliaries meet the requirements of the monographs in the pharmacopoeias that are regarded as mandatory in the countries concerned. The products described in this book meet these requirements (Table 183).

The monograph "Povidone" is in stage 5 to be worldwide harmonized.

Table 183. Excipients of this book covered by pharmacopoeias

Product	Ph.Eur.	USP-NF	J.P./J.P.E.
Povidone K 12	+	+	n. a.
Povidone K 17	+	+	+
Povidone K 25-90	+	+	+
Crospovidone	+	+	+
Copovidone	+	+	+

n.a. = Monograph not available

5.1.1.3
Registrations in individual countries

Pharmaceutical products that contain povidone, crospovidone or copovidone have been registered in all important drug markets like Europa, USA, Japan etc. for parenteral, oral and topical administration.

The following limitations apply to povidone in injectables:

1. Japan
   Up to 2001 Povidone K 12 was only registered in one human injectable, and povidone K 17 in different human preparations.
2. Europe
   The use of povidone in finished parenteral preparations was regulated in Germany by the Federal Health Ministry in 1983 [214]:
   - The K-value must be smaller than 18.
   - The packaging and the package insert of the finished declaration must declare the quantity used.
   - Attention must be drawn to the possibility of accumulation in the organism after frequent administration.
   - For intramuscular administration a maximum of 50 mg of povidone is permitted per individual dose.

Similar regulations also apply in other european countries.

5.1.1.4
Drug Master File (DMF)

Drug Masters Files are only required for the registration of excipients not included in the Pharmacopoeias as monographs. Therefore for povidone, crospovidone and copovidone a DMF is not needed for the registration of a drug containing one of these excipients.

5.1.2
Food

5.1.2.1
General

While there are no such lists for pharmaceutical products, various countries have positive lists regulating the use of auxiliaries in food. These lists include soluble and insoluble polyvinylpyrrolidone, though in some cases only for certain applications.

5.1.2.2
ADI value

In 1987 the World Health Organization (WHO + FAO) specified an Accepted Daily Intake (ADI) value for soluble polyvinylpyrrolidone (povidone) in food of 0–50 mg/kg body weight [372]. For Crospovidone the ADI value is “not specified” and therefore no limit is given for the application in foods [215].

5.1.2.3
Registration of povidone in the Europe and USA

In the European Union soluble polyvinylpyrrolidone having a nominal K-value of 25, 30, or 90 has got the E-number E 1201 for the use in dietary food supplements in (coated) tablet form and in sweetener preparations.

Povidone with an average molecular weight of 40 000 (povidone K 30) is registered for use in the USA in the manufacture of the foods listed in Table 184, subject to certain restrictions [487].

In the USA, povidone with a number average molecular weight of 360 000 (povidone K 90) is permitted for use as a clarifying agent for beer. The amount remaining in the beer must not exceed 10 ppm.

5.1.2.4
Registration status of crospovidone for use in food in different countries

In the European Union insoluble polyvinylpyrrolidone (“polyvinylpolypyrrolidone”) has got the E-number E 1202 for the use in dietary food supplements in (coated) tablet form and in sweetener preparations.

Table 184. Registration of povidone K 30 for use in food in the USA

Food	Purpose	Conditions of use
Wine	Clarifying agent	Residue <60 ppm
Vinegar	Clarifying agent	Residue <40 ppm
Vitamin, mineral or flavouring concentrates in tablet form	Tabletting auxiliary	According to cGMP rules
Sweetener tablets	Tabletting auxiliary	According to cGMP rules
Vitamin and mineral or sweetener concentrates in liquid form	Stabilizer, dispersant, thickener	According to cGMP rules

Crospovidone is usually registered as "polyvinylpolypyrrolidone" or "PVPP" – in the USA for clarifying beverages and vinegar [488] and in all european and many other countries for stabilizing and clarifying beer and wine.

5.2 Toxicological data

5.2.1 Povidone and crospovidone

There are a large number of publications on the good tolerance of polyvinylpyrrolidone [127–129, 131, 133–134, 201, 225]. A complete list with assessments is to be found in "A Critical Review of the Kinetics and Toxicology of Polyvinylpyrrolidone" by Robinson, Sullivan, Borzelleca and Schwartz, published in 1990 [225].

Because of the good tolerance of povidone, its Accepted Daily Intake (ADI) was adjusted to 0–50 mg/kg body weight by the FAO/WHO Joint Expert Committee for Food Additives (JECFA) in 1987 [372].

In 1983, the JECFA awarded crospovidone an ADI status of "not specified", as on the basis of the available chemical, biochemical, toxicological and other data, the entire daily intake of the substance in the quantities to be expected did not represent any risk to health in the opinion of the JECFA. It therefore seemed unnecessary to set a numerical value for the ADI [215].

Many toxicological and biochemical studies have been carried out with the individual grades of povidone and crospovidone by the producers. They could be ordered there.

There is also a published study on renal elimination after intravenous administration of povidone K 12 and K 17 in rats [97].

The following summary of toxicological properties is taken from the book "A Critical Review of the Kinetics and Toxicology of Polyvinylpyrrolidone" [225]:

Toxicology and Safety
An extensive body of toxicological data in animals supports the biological inertness of PVP. The acute, subchronic, and chronic toxicity of orally administered PVP is extremely low, with the only effect observed being diarrhea at high doses due to the osmotic action of PVP acting as a bulk purgative. Occasional observations of minimal absorption with storage in mesenteric lymph nodes seem to be of no toxicological importance. PVP is neither a sensitizer nor an irritant. There are no reported adverse effects following oral administration in humans. The currently permitted FAO/WHO ADI of 0 – 50 mg/kg body weight for food uses provides an adequate margin of safety. There would appear to be no reason to restrict its oral or topical pharmaceutical use or topical cosmetic use in any way. There have been no reports of adverse effects following its use intravenously as a plasma expander, even after the administration of very large amounts. The only toxicological problems have involved the repeated injection of large amounts of the higher molecular weight material into poorly perfused sites such as subcuta-

neously and into the breast. If the use of PVP in injectables for repeated use is restricted to PVP with a molecular weight less than K-18 in limited amounts (e. g. 50 mg/i. m. dose) and the injection sites are varied, and intramuscular or intravenous routes are used, then these problems should not occur. The repeated use of PVP in depot preparations, which could lead to excessive storage, is not to be recommended.

5.2.2
Copovidone

Copovidone has no acute toxicity and does not irritate the skin or mucous membranes. Prolonged administration to rats and dogs was tolerated without recognizable undesirable side effects.

A prenatal toxicity test on rats gave no indication of adverse effects.

Many detailed toxicologiecal studies have been carried out by the producers where they could be ordered.

6 Literature references

[1] R. Vieweg, M. Reiher, H. Scheurlen, Kunststoff-Handbuch XI, 558–569, Carl-Hanser-Verlag, München (1971)

[2] DOS 2255.263 (1974) + US patent 3,933,766 (1976) BASF AG

[3] S. Kornblum, S. Stoopak, J. Pharm. Sci. 62 (1973) 43–49

[4] H. F. Kauffmann, J. W. Breitenbach, Angew. Makromol. Ch. 45 (1975) 167–175

[5] J. W. Breitenbach, IUPAC Symposium Makromol. Ch. Budapest (1967) 529–544

[6] J. W. Breitenbach, H. F. Kauffmann, G. Zwilling, Makromol. Ch. 177 (1976) 2787–2792

[7] S. Keipert, J. Becker, H.-H. Schultze, R. Voigt, Pharmazie 28 No. 3 (1973) 145–183

[8] W. Scholtan, Makromol. Ch. 11 (1953) 131–230

[9] H. U. Schenck, P. Simak, E. Haedicke, J. Pharm. Sci. 68 No. 12 (1979) 1505–1509

[10] D. Guttmann, T. Higuchi, J. Am. Pharm. Assoc. Sci. 45 (1956) 659–664

[11] H. Macionga, Dissertation, Ludwig-Maximilian-Universität München (1964)

[12] Belg. Patent 602.152 (1961) Hoechst AG

[13] H. Fikentscher, Cellulosechemie 13 (1932) 58–64 und 71–74

[14] W. Appel, E. Biekert, Angew. Chemie 80 No. 18 (1968) 719–725

[15] G. B. Levy, H. P. Frank, J. Polymer. Sci. 17 (1955) 247–254

[16] G. V. Schulz, F. Blaschke, J. Prakt. Ch. 158 (1941) 130–135 + G. V. Schulz, G. Sing, J. Prakt. Ch. 161 (1943) 161–180

[17] L. Ehrhardt, Dissertationsschrift Universität Hamburg (1969)

[18] K. Müller, Pharm. Acta Helv. 43 (1968) 107–122

[19] J. Breinlich, Pharm. Ztg. 118 No. 12 (1973) 440–444

[20] H. Wieczorek, Ch. Junge, Deutsche Lebensmittel-Rundschau 68 (1972) 137–139

[21] DAS 2631.780 (1976) BASF AG

[22] GB patent 1.131.007 (1967)

[23] DOS 2001.604 (1970) Pfizer GmbH

[24] H. Junginger, Pharm. Ind. 39 (1977) 383–388 and 498–501

[25] A. Sh. Geneidi, A. A. Ali, R. B. Salama, J. Pharm. Sci. 67 No. 1 (1978) 114–116

[26] DAS 1119.463 (1960) Hoechst AG

[27] Th. R. Bates, J. Pharm. Pharmacol. 21 (1969) 710–712
[28] DAS 1258.527 (1963) Sankyo Ltd.
[29] DAS 1091.287 (1969) Byk Gulden Lomberg GmbH
[30] A. P. Simonelli, S. C. Mehta, W. I. Higuchi, a) J. Pharm. Sci. 58 (1969) 538–549; b) J. Pharm. Sci. 59 (1970) 633–638; c) J. Pharm. Sci. 65 (1976) 355–361
[31] H. Kala, J. Traue, Acta Pharm. Tech. 29 No. 1 (1983) 29–34
[32] J. H. Collett, G. Kesteven, J. Pharm. Pharmacol. 26 Suppl., 84 p–85 p (1974)
[33] H. Matsumaru, S. Tsuchiya, T. Hosono, Chem. Pharm. Bull. 25 No. 10 (1977) 2504–2509
[34] O. I. Corrigan, R. F. Timoney, J. Pharm. Pharmacol. 27, 759–764 (1975)
[35] M. J. Cho, A. G. Mitchell, M. Pernarowski, J. Pharm. Sci. 60 No. 5, 720–724 (1971)
[36] DAS 2634.004 (1976)
[37] W. Schlemmer, F. Stanislaus, K. D. Rehm, Acta Pharm. Tech. 25 No. 2 (1979) 81–91
[38] B. C. Lippold, R. Lütschg, a) Pharm. Ind. 40 No. 5, 541–549 (1978); b) Pharm. Ind. 40 No. 6, 647–653 (1978); c) Acta Pharm. Tech. 24, 213 (1978)
[39] US patent 3,041,239 (1962) Johnson & Johnson
[40] H. Junginger, a) Pharm. Ind. 36 (1974) 100–104; b) Pharm. Ind. 38 (1976) 461–471
[41] G. H. Svoboda, M. J. Sweeney, W. D. Wakling, J. Pharm. Sci. 60 No. 2, 333 (1971)
[42] T. Tachibana, A. Nakamura, Kolloid-Z. + Z. Polym. 203, 130–133 (1965)
[43] Japanese patent 24379 (07.09.59/14.08.79) Takeda Yakuhin Kokyo K. K.
[44] A. A. Kassem, S. A. Zaki, N. M. Mursi, S. A. Tayel, a) Pharmazie, 34 No. 1 (1979) 43–44; b) Pharm. Ind. 41 No. 4 (1979) 390–393; c) Pharm. Ind. 41 No. 12 (1979) 1220–1223
[45] M. Moriyama, A. Inoue, M. Isoya, M. Tanaka, M. Hanano, J. Pharm. Soc. Japan 98 No. 8, 1012–1018 (1978)
[46] E. Nürnberg, Acta Pharm. Tech. 26 No. 1 (1980) 39–67
[47] E. J. Stupak, Th. R. Bates, a) J. Pharm. Sci. 61 (1972) 400–404; b) J. Pharm. Sci. 62 (1973) 1806–1809
[48] M. H. Rutz-Coudray, J. Giust, P. Buri, Pharm. Acta Helv. 54 No. 12 (1979) 363
[49] US patent 3,089,818 (1960) Baxter Labs.
[50] M. Mayersohn, M. Gibaldi, J. Pharm. Sci. 55 (1966) 1323–1324
[51] E. Nürnberg, M. Krieger, Acta Pharm. Tech. 25 No. 1 (1979) 49–63
[52] A. Hoelgaard, N. Möller, a) Arch. Pharm. Chem. Sci. 3 (1975) 34–37; b) Arch. Pharm. Chem. Sci. 3 (1975) 65–72
[53] O. I. Corrigan, R. F. Timoney, M. J. Whelan, J. Pharm. Pharmacol. 28 (1976) 703–706
[54] D. Schenck, Acta Pharm. Tech. 25 No. 4 (1979) 241–281
[55] S. El Gamal, N. Borie, Y. Hammouda, Pharm. Ind. 40 No. 12 (1978) 1373–1376
[56] M. B. Dexter, J. Pharm. Pharmacol. 27 Suppl. (1975) 58 p
[57] D. E. Resetarits, K. C. Cheng, B. A. Bolton, P. N. Prasad, E. Shefter, T. R. Bates, Int. J. Pharm. 2 No. 2 (1979) 113–123

[58] M.X. Cygnus, J. Taw, C.M. Chiang, Int. J. Pharm. 142 No. 1, 115–119 (1996)
[59] E. Nürnberg, Pharm. Ind. 38 (1976) 74–82 and 228–232
[60] DAS 1137.009 (1961) Bayer AG
[61] H. Sekikawa, M. Nakano, T. Arita, Chem. Pharm. Bull. 27 No. 5 (1979) 1223–1230
[62] W. Scholtan, Arzn. - Forschung 14 (1964) 469
[63] S. A. Said, S. F. Saad, Austr. J. Pharm. Sci. 4 (1975) 121–122
[64] H. Seager, Manufacturing Chemist and Aerosol News 48 No. 4 (1977) 25–35
[65] C. F. Harwood, N. Pilpel, J. Pharm. Sci. 57 No. 3 (1968) 478–481
[66] W. C. Davies, W. T. Gloor Jr., J. Pharm. Sci. 61 No. 4 (1972) 618–622
[67] K. A. Khan, C. T. Rhodes, Drug Devel. Commun. 1 No. 6 (1974–1975) 553–556
[68] K. Pintye-Hodi, B. Selmeczi, G. Kevessy, a) Pharm. Ind. 38 No. 10, 926–930 (1976); b) Pharm. Ind. 38 No. 12, 1171–1174 (1976); c) Pharm. Ind. 39 No. 3, 278–281 (1977)
[69] B. Kovacs, M. Gyarmathy, L. Gyarmathy, Acta Pharm. Hung. 47 No. 2 (1977) 81–89
[70] W. Erni, W. A. Ritschel, a) Pharm. Ind. 39 No. 1, 82–84 (1977); b) Pharm. Ind. 39 No. 3, 284–290 (1977); c) Pharm. Ind. 39 No. 7, 708–711 (1977)
[71] E. Ugri-Hunysdvari, Arch. Pharmaz. 308 (1975) 615–622
[72] H. Takenaka, Y. Kawashima, T. Yoneyama, K. Matsuda, Chem. Pharm. Bull. 19 No. 6 (1971) 1234–1244
[73] DOS 2307.747 (1973)
[74] M. Rouiller, R. Gurny, E. Doelker, Acta Pharm. Tech. 21 (1975) 129–138
[75] J. N. C. Healey, M. H. Rubinstein, V. Walters, J. Pharm. Pharmacol. 26 (1974) Suppl. 41 P – 46 P
[76] B. R. Bhutani, V. N. Bhatia, J. Pharm. Sci. 64 No. 1 (1975) 135–139
[77] E. Shotton, N. J. Edwards, J. Pharm. Pharmacol. 26 (1974) Suppl. 107 P
[78] Belg. patent 593354 (1960) Abbott Labs.
[79] E. Rotteglia, Boll. Chim. Farmac. 95 (1956) 238–250
[80] S. Ahsan, S. Blaug, Drug Standards 26 (1958) 29–33
[81] H. Köhler, Dt. Apoth.-Ztg. 102 No. 17, 507–510 (1962)
[82] M. Ahmed, N. Pilpel, Manufacturing Chemist and Aerosol News 38 No. 1 (1967) 37–38
[83] APV, "Ophthalmica I, Pharm. Grundlagen ihrer Zubereitungen", Wiss. Verlagsges., Stuttgart (1975)
[84] T. von Haugwitz, Klin. Mbl. Augenh. 146 (1965) 723–727
[85] U. Münzel, Schweiz. Apoth.-Ztg. 101 (1963) 929
[86] "Polygyl® Ophthalmic Solution", product literature Schieffelin & Co, New York, USA
[87] US patent 3,920,810 (1974) Burton Parsons Inc.
[88] Japanese patent 0126245 (1974) Allergan Pharm. Inc.
[89] R. Hüttenrauch, J. Keiner, Pharmazie 28 (1973) 137
[90] K. A. Khan, D. J. Rooke, Manufacturing Chemist + Aerosol News 47 No. 1 (1976) 25–26

[91] K. A. Khan, D. J. Rooke, a) J. Pharm. Pharmacol. 26 Suppl., 106–107 (1974); b) J. Pharm. Pharmacol. 28 No. 8, 633–636 (1976)
[92] DAS 2647.364; Kukident Krisp GmbH
[93] DOS 2549.740; Sandoz
[94] C. Boymond, D. Gissinger, A. Stamm, Pharm. Acta Helv. 57 No. 5–6, 131–135 (1982)
[95] S. T. Horhota, J. Burgio, L. Lonski, C. T. Rhodes, J. Pharm. Sci. 65 No. 12 (1976) 1746–1749
[96] K. Kinget, R. Kemel, Pharmazie 40 No. 7, 475–478 (1985)
[97] A. Schiller, G. Reb, R. Taugner, Arzn.-Forsch./Drug Res. 28 (II) No. 11 (1978) 2064–2070
[98] DOS 3006.635 (1980) BASF AG
[99] G. Jürgensen, Dissertation "Komplexbildung zwischen Pharmaka und makromolekularen Hilfsstoffen", Zurich (1966)
[100] M. R. Baichwal, B. N. Kale, Indian J. Pharm. Sci. 41 No. 6 (1979) 255
[101] J. Sciuk, Pharm. Ind. 24, 586–588 (1962)
[102] S. Keipert, R. Voigt, R. Karst, R. Nowak, Pharmazie 34 No. 12 (1979) 818–824
[103] S. Keipert, R. Voigt, K. H. Schwarz, Pharmazie 35 No. 1 (1980) 35–40
[104] S. Keipert, R. Voigt, Pharmazie 35 No. 1 (1980) 52
[105] H. O. Ammar, A. A. Kassem, H. A. Salama, M. S. El-Ridy, Pharm. Ind. 42 No. 7 (1980) 757–761
[106] T. Hosono, S. Tsuchiya, H. Matsumaru, a) Chem. Pharm. Bull. 27 (1979) 58–64; b) J. Pharm. Sci. 69 No. 7 (1980) 824–826
[107] Z. T. Chowhan, J. Pharm. Sci. 69 No. 1 (1980) 1–4
[108] K. H. Gustavson, a) Svensk Kem. Tidskr. 66 No. 12 (1954) 359–362; b) Leder 14 (1963) 27–34
[109] DAS 2554.533 (1975) Sandoz-Patent GmbH
[110] DAS 1767.891 (1968) Pfizer GmbH
[111] H. Sekikawa, T. Naganuma, J. Fujiwara, M. Nakano, T. Arita, Chem. Pharm. Bull. 27 No. 1 (1979) 31–37
[112] DAS 2546.371 (1975) Sandoz-Patent GmbH
[113] W. Hespe, Y. J. Blankwater, J. Wieriks, Arzn.-Forsch./Drug Res. 25 No. 10 (1975) 1561–1564
[114] DOS 1617.328 (1966) Boehringer Ingelheim
[115] F. A. Konev, Chim.-Farm. Z., Moskva 10 No. 9 (1976) 123–126
[116] Japanese patent 42347 (1965) Taisho Ltd.
[117] H. Hess, H. J. Janssen, Pharm. Acta Helv. 44 No. 10, 581–601 (1969)
[118] GB patent 1.099.722 (1965) Takeda Ltd.
[119] A. R. Ebian, M. A. Moustafa, S. A. Khalil, M. M. Motawi, J. Pharm. Pharmacol. 25 (1973) 13–20
[120] US patent 2,793,156 (1957) Bristol Labs.
[121] Belg. Patent 747659 (1968) Bristol Myers Co.
[122] Japanese patent 7125024 (1970) Takeda Ltd.
[123] J. E. Hilton, M. P. Summers, a) Int. J. Pharm. 32, 13–19 (1986); b) Int. J. Pharm. 33, 219–224 (1986)

[124] H. A. Shelanski, M. V. Shelanski, J. Internat. Coll. Surgeons 25 (1956) June
[125] DAS 1767.831 (1968) + US patent 3,725,541 (1973) Roussel-Uclaf
[126] J. M. Wilkinson, G. G. Stoner, E. P. Hay, D. B. Witwer, CSMA Proceedings, 40th Midyear Meeting of the Chem. Spec. Manufacturers Ass. Inc. (1953)
[127] S. L. Schwartz, Yakuzaigaku 41 No. 4 (1981) 205–217
[128] J. Lindner, Verh. Deutsch. Ges. Path. 44 (1960) 272
[129] A. H. Bronnsack, Pharm. Ind. 38 No. 12 (1976) 1181–1185
[130] I. Ericsson, L. Ljunggren, J. Anal. Appl. Pyrolysis 17 No. 3, 251–260 (1990)
[131] L. W. Burnette, Proceedings Sci. Sect. Toil. Goods Ass. 38 Dec. (1962) 1–4
[132] G. Surén, Acta Pharm. Suecica 7, 483–490 (1970)
[133] D. Scheffner, Inaugural Dissertation, Heidelberg (1955)
[134] W. Wessel, M. Schoog, E. Winkler, Arzn.-Forsch./Drug. Res. 21 (1971) 1468
[135] I. Sugimoto, A. Kuchiki, H. Nakagawa, Chem. Pharm. Bull. 29 No. 6 (1981) 1715–1723
[136] S. Bogdanova, N. Lambov, E. Minkov, Pharm. Ind. 42 No. 11 (1980) 1143–1145
[137] I. Sugimoto, H. Nakagawa, K. Tongo, S. Kondo, I. Iwane, K. Tagahashi, Drug Dev. Ind. Pharm. 6 No. 2 (1980) 137–160
[138] A. A. Badawi, A. A. El Sayed, J. Pharm. Sci. 69 No. 5 (1980) 492–497
[139] P. Esposito, D. Lombardi, L. Boltri, T. Canal, L. Dobetti, Boll. Chim. Farm. 134 No. 3, 122–125 (1995)
[140] H. M. Sadek, J. L. Olsen, Pharm. Tech. 5 No. 2 (1981) 40–48
[141] Ullmanns Encyclopädie der technischen Chemie, 4. Auflage (1980) Band 19, 385–390
[142] T. M. Riedhammer, J. Ass. Off. Anal. Chem. 62 No. 1 (1979) 52–55
[143] A. G. E. Pearse, Histochem. Theoret. Appl. (1961) 948
[144] D. G. Freiman, E. A. Gall, Am. J. Clin. Path. 25 (1955) 1427–1429
[145] H. Sekikawa, M. Nakano, T. Arita, Yakugaku Zasshi 98 No. 1 (1978) 62–66
[146] N. Lambov, S. Bogdanova, E. Minkov, Pharm. Ind. 43 No. 5 (1981) 489–491
[147] H. Suzuki et al., Chem. Pharm. Bull. 44, 2, 364–371 (1996)
[148] H. P. Merkle, a) Pharm. Ind. 42 No. 10, 1009–1018 (1980); b) Acta Pharm. Tech. 27, 193–203 (1981); c) Pharm. Acta Helv. 57, 160–163 (1982)
[149] H. P. Merkle, a) Pharm. Ind. 43 No. 2 (1981) 183–188; b) Pharm. Ind. 43 No. 4 (1981) 380–388
[150] H. Sekikawa, M. Nakano, M. Takada, T. Arita, Chem. Pharm. Bull. 28 No. 8 (1980) 2443–2449
[151] D. E. Cadwallader, D. K. Madan, J. Pharm. Sci. 70 No. 4 (1981) 442–446
[152] K. Takayama, N. Nambu, T. Nagai, a) Chem. Pharm. Bull. 28 No. 11 (1980) 3304–3309; b) Chem. Pharm. Bull. 29 No. 9 (1981) 2718–2721
[153] A. Ghanem, M. Meshali, I. Ramadaan, Pharmazie 35 No. 11 (1980) 689–690
[154] E. C. Lipman, M. P. Summers, J. Pharm. Pharmacol. 32 Suppl. 21 P (1980)
[155] S. Bogdanova, N. Lambov, E. Minkov, Pharm. Ind. 43 No. 7 (1981) 679–681
[156] S. Kocova El-Arini, Pharm. Ind. 43 No. 7 (1981) 674–679
[157] J. Varshosaz, R. A. Kennedy, E. M. Gipps, Drug. Dev. Ind. Pharm. 23 No. 6, 611–618 (1997)
[158] K. H. Frömming, W. Ditter, D. Horn, J. Pharm. Sci. 70 No. 7 (1981) 738–743

[159] H. Kala, J. Traue, H. Moldenhauer, G. Zessin, Pharmazie 36 No. 2 (1981) 106–111

[160] D. Essig, P. Schmidt, H. Stumpf, W. A. P. Luck, "Flüssige Arzneiformen und Arzneimittelsicherheit", 38–42 + 47, Wiss. Verlagsgesellschaft mbH, Stuttgart (1981)

[161] E. Nürnberg, M. Krieger, Pharm. Ind. 43 No. 8 (1981) 786–791

[162] R. Voigt, D. Terborg, Pharmazie 35 No. 5/6 (1980) 311–312

[163] US patent 4,018,889 (1977) Pfizer Inc.

[164] Eur. patent 0.021.847 (1980) Pfizer Inc.

[165] S. Bogdanova, N. Lambow, E. Minkow, a) Pharmazie 36 No. 6 (1981) 415–416; b) Pharmazie 37 No. 3 (1982) 197–19

[166] S. K. Podder, K. C. Moy, V. H. L. Lee, Exp. Eye Res. 54, 747–757 (1992)

[167] E. Nürnberg, G. Bleimüller, Pharm. Ind. 43 No. 6 (1981) 570–571

[168] S. S. Kornblum, B. Lopez, J. Pharm. Sci. 59 No. 7 (1970) 1016–1018

[169] DOS 1667.924 (1968) + DOS 1811.810 (1968)

[170] DAK-Praeparater 1963 (01.04.65), 781, Denmark

[171] DAK-Vorschrift, Arch. Pharm. og Chem. 73 (1966) 244–245

[172] H. Köhler, J. Österreich, B. Quarck, Dt. Apoth.-Ztg. 102, 1–8 (1962)

[173] K. Münzel, Pharm. Acta Helv. 38 (1963) 65–85 + 129–146

[174] DAS 2021.786 (1970), Colorcon Inc.

[175] US patent 3,524,756 (1967) Colorcon Inc.

[176] A. S. Alam, E. L. Parrott, J. Pharm. Sci. 61 No. 2 (1972) 265–268

[177] A. Dommeyer, I. Baucherat, P. Buri, Acta Pharm. Tech. 27 No. 4 (1981) 205–210

[178] Sang-Chue Shin, Arch. Pharm. Res. 2 No. 1 (1979) 35–47 + 49–64

[179] J. A. Plaizier-Vercammen, R. E. De Nève, a) J. Pharm. Sci. 69 No. 12, 1403–1408 (1980); b) J. Pharm. Sci. 70, 1252–1256 (1981); c) J. Pharm. Sci. 71 No. 5, 552–556 (1982); d) J. Pharm. Sci. 72 No. 9, 1042–1044 (1980)

[180] E. Graf, Ch. Beyer, O. Abdallah, a) Acta Pharm. Tech. 28 No. 2, 131–135 (1982); b) Acta Pharm. Tech. 28 No. 3, 225–230 (1982)

[181] K. Kono, T. Nagai, H. Nogami, Chem. Pharm. Bull. 18 No. 6 (1970) 1287–1288

[182] Eur. patent 0.003.682 (1982) Merck & Co Inc.

[183] M. A. Attia, A. E. Aboutaleb, F. S. Habib, Pharmazie 37 No. 4, 274–277 (1982)

[184] H. Sekikawa, J. Fujiwara, T. Naganuma, M. Nakano, T. Arita, Chem. Pharm. Bull. 26 No. 10 (1978) 3033–3039

[185] Eur. patent 0.012.495 + 0.012.496 (1979), Beecham Group Ltd.

[186] DAS 1028.741 (1956), Leybold GmbH

[187] L. Krowczynski, Pharmazie 37 No. 1 (1982) 79–83

[188] M. A. Kassem, A. E. El-Nimr, S. M. Omar, Pharmazie 37 No. 4 (1982) 280–281

[189] N. K. Patel et al., Proceed. Int. Symp. Contr. Rel. Bioact. Mater. 23, 147–148 (1996)

[190] A. M. Motawi, S. A. M. Mortadu, F. El Khawas, K. A. El Khodery, Acta Pharm. Tech. 28 No. 3 (1982) 211–215

[191] K. D. Bremecker, Acta Pharm. Tech. 28 No. 3 (1982) 199–206

[192] D. Horn, W. Ditter, J. Pharm. Sci. 71 No. 9 (1982) 1021–1026

[193] DAS 1617.576 (1967), Gisten Spiritusfabriek N.
[194] H. Sekikawa, N. Yagi, J. Sakuragi, K. Tanaka, M. Sakamoto, M. Itoh, M. Takada, T. Arita, Chem. Pharm. Bull. 30 No. 2 (1982) 739–74
[195] K. Takayama, N. Nambu, T. Nagai, Chem. Pharm. Bull. 30 No. 2 (1982) 673–678
[196] K. Takayama, N. Nambu, T. Nagai, Chem. Pharm. Bull. 30 No. 8 (1982) 3013–3016
[197] J. C. Callahan, G. W. Cleary, M. Elefant, G. Kaplan, T. Kensler, R. A. Nash, Drug Dev. Ind. Pharm. 8 No. 3 (1982) 355–369
[198] DOS 1924.647 (1969), Sanol-Schwarz GmbH
[199] E. James, K. C. Varma, S. N. Sharma, Indian J. Pharm. Sci. 45 No. 1 (1983) 52
[200] N. A. El-Gindy, A. H. Karara, M. M. Abd El-Khalek, Sci. Pharm. 44 No. 4 (1976) 315–322
[201] P. Knolle, Pharm. Ind. 44 No. 9 (1982) 865–874
[202] L. J. Frauenfelder, J. of A. O. A. C. 57 No. 4 (1974) 796–800
[203] T. Jira, B. Panzig, Pharmazie 37 No. 8 (1980) 587–590
[204] A. E. Dobrotvorsky, S. M. Vyrovshchikova, Farmatsiya 31 No. 6 (1982) 42–45
[205] I. Sugimoto, K. Sasaki, A. Kuchiki, T. Ishihava, H. Nakagawa, Chem. Pharm. Bull. 30 No. 12 (1982) 4479–4488
[206] S. S. El Dalsh, A. A. El-Sayed, A. A. Badawi, A. Fouli, Pharmazie 37 No. 8 (1982) 606–607
[207] K. Takayama, H. Imaizumi, N. Nambu, T. Nagai, a) Chem. Pharm. Bull. 30 No. 10, 3701–3710 (1982); b) J. Pharm. Dyn. 5, S 3 (1982); c) Chem. Pharm. Bull. 31, 4496–4507 (1983)
[208] N. A. El-Gindy, A. A. Shalaby, M. M. A. El-Khalek, Drug Dev. Ind. Pharm. 9 No. 6 (1983) 1031–1045
[209] H. Sekikawa, N. Fukuda, M. Takada, K. Obtani, T. Arita, M. Nakano, Chem. Pharm. Bull. 31 No. 4 (1983) 1350–1356
[210] A. Esteve, A. del Pozo, P. J. Solanas, R. Salazar, Cienc. Ind. Farm. 2 No. 5 (1983) 175–183
[211] A. Palmieri, T. Danson, W. Groben, R. Jukka, C. Dummer, Drug Dev. Ind. Pharm. 9 No. 3 (1983) 421–442
[212] V. Bühler, U. Klodwig, Acta Pharm. Tech. 30 No. 4, 317–324 (1984)
[213] R. Tawashi, a) Drugs Made in Germ. 8, 178–184 (1965); b) Pharm. Ind. 26, 682–685 (1964)
[214] Bundesanzeiger No. 123 (1983) 6666
[215] FAO/WHO-Report No. 27 (1983) 26–27
[216] H. V. van Kamp, G. K. Bolhuis, C. F. Lerk, Pharm. Weekblad Sci. Ed. 5 (1983) 165–171
[217] V. Bühler, US-Pharmacopeial Forum, May – June 1984, 4287–4289
[218] K.-F. Jäger, K. H. Bauer, Acta Pharm. Technol. 30 No. 1 (1984) 85–92
[219] H. Junginger, M. Wedler, Acta Pharm. Technol. 30 No. 1 (1984) 68–77
[220] J. A. Plaizier-Vercammen, J. Pharm. Sci. 72 No. 9 (1983) 1042–1044

[221] C. Caramella, P. Colombo, G. Bettinetti, F. Giordano, Acta Pharm. Tech. 30 No. 2 (1984) 132–139
[222] H. Imaizumi, N. Nambu, T. Nagai, Chem. Pharm. Bull. 31 No. 7 (1983) 2510–2512
[223] A. Matthes, Angew. Chemie 54, 517 (1941)
[224] R. Iwaoku, Y. Okamatsu, S. Kino, K. Arimori, M. Nakano, Chem. Pharm. Bull. 32 No. 3 (1984) 1091–1095
[225] B. V. Robinson, F. M. Sullivan, J. F. Borzelleca, S. L. Schwartz, "PVP – A Critical Review of the Kinetics and Toxicology of Polyvinylpyrrolidone (Povidone)", Lewis Publishers (1990)
[226] Y. Nozawa, T. Mizumoto, F. Higashide, Pharm. Acta Helv. 60 No. 5–6 (1985) 175–177
[227] S. Keipert, Pharmazie 39 No. 9 (1984) 644–647
[228] S. E. Leucuta, R. D. Pop, A. Grasu, C. Georgescu, F. Gitlan, Farmacia (Bukarest) 32 No. 1 (1984) 27–34
[229] I. Popovici, E. Gafitanu, E. Stefanescu, V. Dorneanu, I. Vasiliu, Farmacia (Bukarest) 32 No. 1 (1984) 13–20
[230] E. Gafitanu, I. Popovici, E. Stefanescu, V. Dorneanu, M. Vasilescu, Farmacia (Bukarest) 32 No. 1 (1984) 21–26
[231] E. Nürnberg, Pharm. Ind. 28 No. 5 (1966) 291–304
[232] F. Carli, F. Garbassi, J. Pharm. Sci. 74 No. 9 (1985) 963–967
[233] A. V. Deshpande, D. K. Agrawal, Drug Dev. Ind. Pharm. 10 No. 10 (1984) 1725–1736
[234] A. V. Deshpande, D. K. Agrawal, Pharmazie 40 No. 7 (1985) 496–497
[235] A. Urtti, L. Perviviita, L. Salminen, M. Juslin, Drug Dev. Ind. Pharm. 11 No. 2 + 3 (1985) 257–268
[236] O. I. Corrigan, E. M. Holohan, M. R. Reilly, Drug Dev. Ind. Pharm. 11 No. 2 + 3 (1985) 677–695
[237] DOS 3228.384 (1982) Rentschler Arzneimittel
[238] J. L. Ford, Pharm. Acta Helv. 61 No. 3 (1986) 69–88
[239] A. M. Guyot-Hermann, D. Leblanc, M. Draguet-Brughmans, Drug Dev. Ind. Pharm. 11 No. 2 + 3 (1985) 551–564
[240] Patents, Bayer AG, a) DOS 3424.553 (1984); b) Eur. Patent 0078.430 (1982); c) Eur. Patent 0167.909 (1985)
[241] L. S. C. Wan, Y. L. Choong, Pharm. Acta Helv. 61 No. 5–6 (1986) 150–156
[242] D. I. Dmitrievsky, A. I. Maslennikov, V. N. Vidashenko, L. F. Checherskaya, Farm. Zh. (Kiev) No. 4, 52–55 (1985)
[243] P. L. Gould, S. B. Tan, Drug Dev. Ind. Pharm. 11 No. 2–3 (1985) 441–460
[244] I. Sugimoto, T. Ishihara, H. Habata, H. Nakagawa, J. Parew Sci. Tech. 35 No. 3 (1981) 88–92
[245] GB patent 792,544 (1965), American Home Corp.
[246] Fr. patent 011 589 (1969) = Belg. patent 748 897 (1970) Orsymonde S. A.
[247] F. Gstirner, G. Said, Pharm. Ind. 10 (1971) 683–685
[248] DP 940134 (1951) Bayer AG
[249] H. Helle, Pharm. Ind. 24 No. 11 a (1962) 550–553

[250] J. A. Plaizier-Vercammen, C. Bruwier, Sci. Tech. Prak. Pharm. 2 No. 17 (1986) 525–530

[251] Y. Nozawa, T. Mizumoto, F. Higashide, Pharm. Acta Helv. 61 No. 12 (1986) 337–341

[252] H. Kala, U. Haack, F. Fahr, P. Pollandt, Pharmazie 41 No. 1 (1986) 61–62

[253] M. Sumnu, S.T.P. Pharma 2 No. 14 (1986) 214–220

[254] S. Keipert, R. Voigt, Pharmazie 41 No. 6 (1986) 400–404

[255] N. M. Najib, M. Suleiman, A. Malakh, Int. J. Pharmaceutics 32, 229–236 (1986)

[256] Eur. Patent 0.212.853 (1986) Warner Lambert Group

[257] US patent 3,988,439 (1976) Eli Lilly Corp.

[258] C. Doherty, P. York, J. Pharm. Sci. 76 No. 9 (1987) 731–737

[259] J. Akbuga, A. Gürsoy, E. Kendi, Drug Dev. Ind. Pharm. 14 No. 10 (1988) 1439–1464

[260] Y. Takahashi, T. Trukuda, Ch. Izumi et al., Chem. Pharm. Bull. 36 No. 7 (1988) 2708–2710

[261] M. A. Kassem, M. S. El-Ridy, L. M. Khairy, Drug Dev. Ind. Pharm. 13 No. 7 (1987) 1171–1196

[262] H. V. van Kamp, G. K. Bolhuis, C. F. Lerk, Acta Pharm. Suecica 23, 217–230 (1986)

[263] DAS 2950.154 (1989) Sandoz

[264] G. P. Bettini, P. Mura, A. Liquori, G. Bramanti, Il Farmaco Ed. Pr. 43, 11 (1988) 331–343

[265] C. Doherty, P. York, Drug Dev. Ind. Pharm. 15 No. 12 (1989) 1969–1987

[266] A. Abd El-Bary et al., Drug Dev. Ind. Pharm. 16 No. 10, 1649–1660 (1990)

[267] C.-H. Chiang, S.-J. Chang, Advances Pharm. Tech. (1989) 142–151

[268] H. Nakagawa, Advances Pharm. Tech. (1989) 203–211

[269] US patent 4,851,543 (1988) GAF Corp.

[270] Y. Il Kim, J. Pharm. Soc. Korea, Vol. 23 No. 2, 81–94 (1979)

[271] F. Carli, I. Colombo, L. Rabaglia, F. Borella, Poster Session, Congresso AFI, Salsomaggiore, May 1990

[272] R. Bianchini, C. Torricelli, C. Vecchio, Acta Tech. Leg. Med. 1 No. 8, 57–72 (1990)

[273] J. van Niekerk, S. I. Pather, I. Russell, Poster Session, Academy of Pharm. Sciences, Congress, South Africa, 24.–26.04.90

[274] S. Richard, J. Paris, J. H. Aiache, J. Couquelet, Biopharm. Pharmacokinet. Eur. Congr. 2d. 1, 288–297 (1984)

[275] Y. K. Agrawal, K. Prakasam, J. Pharm. Sci. 77 No. 10, 885–888 (1988)

[276] Eur. patent 0.339.506, Ciba Geigy (1989)

[277] N. M. Najib, M. A. El-Hinnawi, M. S. Suleiman, Pharm. Res. 5 No. 10, 141 (1988)

[278] Eur. patent 0.342.879, Cryopharm (1989)

[279] US patent 4,863,724, Thomae (1989)

[280] DE 3413.955, Sandoz (1984)

[281] US patent 4,851,226, McNeil Consumer Prod. (1989)

[282] Int. patent PCT WO 89/07520 + 07521, Bristol-Myers (1989)
[283] E. M. Ramadan et al., Bull. Pharm. Sci., Assiut Univ. 9, 30–49 (1986)
[284] E. M. Ramadan et al., Pharm. Ind. 49, 508–513 (1987)
[285] K. M., O'Driscoll, O. I. Corrigan, Drug Dev. Ind. Pharm. 8, 547–564 (1982)
[286] M. H. Rutz-Coudray, P. Buri, Congr. Int. Technol. Pharm. 1st, 4, 98–103 (1977)
[287] C. Doherty et al., J. Pharm. Pharmacol. 38, 48P (1986)
[288] East German patent DD 249,186; J. Traue et al.
[289] Ye Huang et al., Yaoxue Xuebao 20, 918–922 (1985); ref. CA 104.230317
[290] A. Kuchiki et al., Yakuzaigaku 44, 31–37 (1984); ref. Int. Pharm. Abstr. 2301271
[291] M. Morita, S. Hirota, Chem. Pharm. Bull. 33, 2091–2097 (1985)
[292] N. Udupa et al., Ind. J. Hosp. Pharm. 23, 268–272 (1986)
[293] S. Sakurai et al., Yakuzaigaku 47, 191–196 (1987)
[294] A. L. Thakkar et al., J. Pharm. Pharmacol. 29, 783–784 (1977)
[295] Japanese patent 79 46,837 Kanebo Ltd.; ref. CA 91.112451
[296] D. Essig, H. Stumpf "Flüssige Arzneiformen schwerlöslicher Arzneistoffe" Chapter VIII (V. Bühler) "Entwicklung von Trockensäften und Trinkgranulaten" Wiss. Verlagsgesellschaft, Stuttgart (1990)
[297] I. Sugimoto et al., Drug Dev. Ind. Pharm. 6, 137–160 (1980)
[298] Japanese patent 81 68,619 Yamanouchi Pharmac. Co.; ref. CA 95.138628
[299] Japanese patent 82 85,316 Kanebo Ltd.; ref. CA 97.78923
[300] A. A. Ali, A. S. Gorashi, Int. J. Pharm. 19, 297–306 (1984)
[301] E. Minkov et al., Farmatsiya (Sofia) 32, 27–29 (1982); ref. CA 97.133483
[302] H. Robert, M. Brazier, Biopharm. Pharmacokinet. Eur. Congr. 2nd 1, 99–108 (1984)
[303] M. Brazier, H. Robert, J. Pharm. Clin. 4, 203 (1985)
[304] S. Yakou et al., Chem. Pharm. Bull. 34, 3408–3414 (1986)
[305] E. I. Stupak et al., J. Pharmacok. Biopharm. 2, 511–524 (1974)
[306] H. Sekikawa et al., Yakugaku Zasshi 98, 62 (1978)
[307] A. V. Deshpande, D. K. Agrawal, Pharmazie 38, 539–541 (1983)
[308] S. A. Ibrahim, S. Shawky, Expo.-Congr. Int. Technol. Pharm. 3rd 5, 203–210 (1983)
[309] Japanese patent 58,206,533 Teijin Ltd.; ref. CA 100.91354
[310] K. Thoma, F. Knott, Pharm. Ztg., Wiss. 2, 179 (1989)
[311] J. H. Dopper et al., abstract FIP congress, page 33 (1977)
[312] A. Witzel, Dissertation Freie Universität Berlin (1988)
[313] B. R. Hajratwala, D. S. S. Ho, J. Pharm. Sci. 73, 1539–1541 (1984)
[314] L. S. C. Wan, K. S. Lim, Sci. Tech. Prat. Pharm. 6 No. 8, 567–573 (1990)
[315] Belg. Patent BE 894,942 Elan Corp. Ltd.; ref. CA 99.76892
[316] O. I. Corrigan, E. M. Holohan, J. Pharm. Pharmacol. 36, 217–221 (1984)
[317] F. Fahr et al., Pharmazie 41, 517 (1986)
[318] S. Bogdanova, N. G. Lamov, E. C. Minkov, Pharm. Ind. 45, 1011–1013 (1983)
[319] H. E. Junginger, M. Wedler, Pharm. Res. 3, 41–44 (1986)

[320] E. M. Ramadan et al., Pharm. Ind. 51, 1293–1296 (1989)
[321] B. Novosel, M. Palka, Farm. Vestn. (Ljubljana) 38, 13–16 (1987); ref. CA 107.161575
[322] M. Sumnu, Sci. Tech. Prat. Pharm. 2, 299–302 (1986)
[323] K. R. P. Shenoy, P. P. Thampi, Indian Drugs 22, 423–426 (1985)
[324] M. Murray, A. Laohavichien, W. Habib, A. Sakr, Pharm. Ind. 60 No. 3, 257–262 (1998)
[325] L. Boltri, N. Coceani, D. Del Curto, L. Dobetti, P. Esposito, Pharm. Dev. Techn. 2 No. 4, 373–381 (1997)
[326] R. Jachowicz, Int. J. Pharm. 35, 7–12 (1987)
[327] Japanese patent 6377,821, Teikoku Seiyaku Co. (1986); ref. CA 109.176362 (1988)
[328] N. Udupa et al., Indian Drugs 23, 221–224 (1986)
[329] C. Wu, J. Tang, Yaoxue Tongbao, 16, 632 (1981); ref. CA 97.28490
[330] N. Udupa et al., Indian Drugs 23, 294 (1986); ref. CA 105.29922
[331] J. Guo, X. Liu, Yaoxue Tongbao 21, 261 (1986); ref. CA 106.9316
[332] Japanese patent 60 64,920 Mitsui Pharmaceuticals, Inc.; ref. CA 103.92837
[333] S. Bogdanova et al., Farmatsiya (Sofia) 31, 25 (1981); ref. CA 96.223095
[334] R. Yan, K. Xia, Zhongcaoyao 19, 492 (1988); ref. CA 110.121204
[335] K. Y. Xia, J. Z. Lu, Chin. Trad. Herbal Drugs 18, 108 (1987); ref. Int. Pharm. Abstr. 2509780 + CA 107.102527
[336] A. S. Geneidi et al., J. Drug Res. Egypt 18 No. 1–2, 29–36 (1989)
[337] DOS 2145.325 Sandoz
[338] D. I. Dmitrievskii, M. Pertsev, Farm. Zh. (Kiev) No. 5, 48–51 (1984); ref. CA 102.32075
[339] A. S. Geneidi et al., Can. J. Pharm. Sci. 15, 81 (1981); ref. CA 95.30290
[340] E. Nürnberg et al., Pharm. Ind. 38, 907 (1976)
[341] O. I. Corrigan, E. M. Holohan, Abstract FIP 127 (1983)
[342] N. M. Najib et al., Int. J. Pharm. 45, 139–144 (1988)
[343] I. Popovici et al., Rev. Chim. (Bucharest) 32, 1059 (1981); ref. CA 96.168652
[344] N. H. Brown, Drug Dev. Ind. Pharm. 4, 427 (1978)
[345] N. Fukuda et al., Chem. Pharm. Bull. 34, 1366 (1986)
[346] M. Kata et al., Acta Pharm. Hung. 54, 210 (1984); ref. Int. Pharm. Abstr. 2205433
[347] E. Minkow et al., Farmatsiya (Sofia) 32, 38 (1982)
[348] G. I. Abdel-Rahman, A. M. El-Sayed, A. E. Aboutaleb, Bull. Pharm. Sci. 11 No. 2 (1989) 261–272
[349] A. K. Singla, T. Vijan, Drug Dev. Ind. Pharm. 16 No. 5 (1990) 875–882
[350] Y. Nozawa et al., Kobunshi Ronbunshu 41 No. 5 (1984) 307–310
[351] Y. Nozawa et al., Kobunshi Ronbunshu 42 No. 11 (1985) 825–828
[352] T. Mizumoto et al., Yakuzaigaku 45 (1985) 291–297
[353] Japanese patent 2015026 (1990) Takeda
[354] Japanese patent 1294620 (1989) Kissei
[355] US patent 4,898,728 (1990) Beecham Group
[356] US patent 4,920,145 (1990) GAF = Internat. Patent 8,907,941 (1989)

[357] I. Orienti, V. Zecchi, C. Cavallari, A. Fini, Acta Pharm. Tech. 36 No. 1 (1990) 11–14
[358] J. L. Vila Jato, C. Remunan, R. Martinez, S.T.P. Pharma 6 No. 2 (1990) 88–92
[359] H.-L. Fung, M. J. Cho, J. Pharm. Sci. 67, 971–975 (1978)
[360] DE 3920.626, Glaxo Paris (1989)
[361] Eur. J. Drug Metab. Pharmacokinet. 15 No. 2 Suppl. (1990) Abstr. 311
[362] G. D. D'Alonzo, R. E. O'Connor, J. B. Schwartz, Drug Dev. Ind. Pharm. 16 No. 12 (1990) 1931–1944
[363] US patent 3,673,163 Eli Lilly USA (1972)
[364] Eur. patent 0.364.944, Vectorpharma (1989)
[365] Eur. patent 0.371.431, Vectorpharma (1989)
[366] A. H. El-Assasy, M. A. A. Kassem, M. I. Mohamed, Bull. Fac. Pharm. Cairo, 27 No. 1, 77–82 (1989)
[367] Eur. patent 0.186.090 + US patent 4,800,086, BASF AG (1985)
[368] V. Bühler, "Vademecum for Vitamin Formulations", Wiss. Verlagsgesellschaft, Stuttgart, Germany (2nd edition, 2001), a) Page 125; b) Page 40; c) Page 62; d) Page 76; e) Pages 76, 80, 99, 102, 105; f) Page 32
[369] DOS 3447.423, BASF AG (1984)
[370] S. K. Bajeva, K. C. Jindal, Ind. J. Pharm. Sci. 14 (1979) 20–24
[371] A. Chapiro, C. Legris, Eur. Polym. J. 1 (1985) 49–53
[372] WHO Technical Report Series 751, FAO/WHO Report No. 30, 30–31 (1987)
[373] J. Wieriks, H. E. Schornagel, Chemotherapy 16 (1971) 85–108
[374] A. Immelman, W. S. Botha, D. Grib, J. S. Afr. Vet. Assoc. 49, No. 2 (1978) 103–105
[375] DOS 3228.335 (1984)
[376] Eur. patent 0.192.173 BASF AG (1986)
[377] M. de Vos, J. M. Kozak, J. van Damme, Proceedings of the 2nd Int. Symp. on Povidone, University of Kentucky, Lexington 1987, 10–23
[378] Japanese patent 1168619 (1989)
[379] DOS 2546.577, Sandoz GmbH (1977)
[380] K. Baba, Y. Takeichi, Y. Nakai, Chem. Pharm. Bull. 38 No. 9 (1990) 2542–2546
[381] Japanese patent 2204497 (1990)
[382] DE 3825.317 (1990) Hausmann A. G.
[383] GB patent 2.218.905 (1989) + US patent 4,917,899 (1990) Elan Corp.
[384] Eur. patent 0.054.279 (1982) Forest Inc.
[385] US patent 4,542,613 (1985), Key Inc. + Int. patent 83.00.093 (1983)
[386] R. Ananthanarayanan, H. L. Bhalla, Indian J. Pharma. Sci. 49 No. 4 (1987) 166
[387] E. Dargel, J. B. Mielck, Acta Pharm. Tech. 35 No. 4, 197–209 (1989)
[388] V. A. Li, P. V. Zinovev, S. Sh. Rashidova, Uzb. Khim. Zh. 3, 49–50 (1990)
[389] K. H. Ziller, H. H. Rupprecht, Pharm. Ind. 52 No. 8, 1017–1022 (1990)
[390] D. Hennig, E. Schubert, Pharmazie 42 No. 11 (1987) 725–728
[391] C. Caramella, F. Ferrari, M. C. Bonferoni, M. Ronchi, Drug Dev. Ind. Pharm. 16 No. 17, 2561–2577 (1990)
[392] D. Gissinger, A. Stamm, Pharm. Ind. 42 No. 2, 189–192 (1980)

[393] H. V. van Kamp, G. K. Bolhuis, C. F. Lerk, Acta Pharm. Tech. 34 No. 1, 11–16 (1989)
[394] H. V. van Kamp, G. K. Bolhuis, C. F. Lerk, et al., Pharm. Acta Helv. 61 No. 1, 22–29 (1986)
[395] P. H. List, U. A. Muazzam, Pharm. Ind. 41, 459–464 (1979)
[396] E. M. Rudnic, C. T. Rhodes, J. F. Bavitz, J. B. Schwartz, Drug Dev. Ind. Pharm. 7 No. 3, 347–358 (1981)
[397] M. Jovanovic, Z. Samardzic, Z. Djuric, L. Zivanovic, Pharmazie 43 No. 10 727 (1988)
[398] C. Caramella, F. Ferrari, U. Conte et al., Acta Pharm. Tech. 35 No. 1, 30–33 (1989)
[399] P. Colombo, U. Conte, C. Caramella, M. Geddo, A. La Manna, J. Pharm. Sci. 73, 701 (1984)
[400] M. Niskanen, J. K. Yliruusi, T. Niskanen, Acta Pharm. Fenn. 99, 129–140 (1990)
[401] K. Takayama, H. Imaizumi, N. Nambu, T. Nagai, Chem. Pharm. Bull. 33, 292–300 (1985)
[402] R. A. Miller, G. R. B. Down, C. H. Yates, J. F. Millar, Can. J. Pharm. Sci. 15 No. 3, 55–58 (1980)
[403] M. S. Gordon, Z. T. Chowhan, Drug Dev. Ind. Pharm. 16 No. 3,437–447 (1990)
[404] J. Gillard, Acta Pharm. Tech. 26 No. 4, 290–292 (1980)
[405] P.-C. Sheen, S.-I. Kim, Drug Dev. Ind. Pharm. 15 No. 3, 401–414 (1989)
[406] S. A. Botha, A. P. Lötter, a) Drug Dev. Ind. Pharm. 15 No. 11, 1843–1853 (1989); b) Drug Dev. Ind. Pharm. 16 No. 4, 673–683 (1990); c) Drug Dev. Ind. Pharm. 16 No. 12, 1945–1954 (1990)
[407] N. A. El-Gindy, M. A. El-Egakey, Sci. Pharm. 49, 427–434 (1981)
[408] M. A. El-Egakey, N. A. El-Gindy, Sci. Pharm. 49, 434–441 (1981)
[409] M. A. El-Egakey, Acta Pharm. Tech. 28 No. 4, 267–271 (1982)
[410] N. Salib, S. Abd El-Fattah, M. El-Massik, Pharm. Ind. 45 No. 9, 902–906 (1983)
[411] P. I. Fekete, Sci. Pharm. 54 No. 3, 168 (1986)
[412] A. R. Patel, M. S. Treki, R. C. Vasavada, J. Controll. Rel. 7 No. 2, 133–138 (1988)
[413] M. R. Baichwal, S. G. Deshande, P. K. Singh, Indian J. Pharm. Sci. 50 No. 3, 153–156 (1988)
[414] US-Patent 5, 676, 968 (1995) Schering
[415] M. R. Baichwal, V. Padma, Indian J. Pharm. Sci. 46 No. 1, 58 (1984)
[416] P. K. Singh, P. Venkitachaiam, M. R. Baichwal, S. G. Deshpande, Indian J. Pharm. Sci. 49 No. 3, 129 (1987)
[417] H. L. Bhalla, R. D. Toddywala, Drug. Dev. Ind. Pharm. 14 No. 1, 119–131 (1988)
[418] S. Gadkari, H. L. Bhalla, Indian J. Pharm. Sci. 48 No. 5, 150 (1986)
[419] Fr. patent 2042326 (1969) Italfarmaco SpA.
[420] R. Salazar, A. del Pozo, Galenica Acta 17, 165–179 (1964)

[421] C.-M. Ma, C.-L. Li, Colloids and Surfaces 47, 117–123 (1990)
[422] H. Gucluyildiz, F. W. Goodhart, J. Pharm. Sci. 66 No. 2, 265–266 (1977)
[423] M. J. Pikal, A. L. Lukes, L. F. Ellis, J. Pharm. Sci. 65 No. 9, 1278–1284 (1976)
[424] B. Vennat, D. Gross, A. Pourrat, P. Legret, J. Pharm. Belg. 48 No. 6, 430–436 (1993)
[425] Y. B. Jun, B. H. Min, S. I. Kim, Y. I. Kim, J. Kor. Pharm. Sci. 19 No. 3, 123–128 (1989)
[426] R. Voigt, G. Thomas, M. Götte, Pharmazie 40 No. 1, 39–44 (1985)
[427] J. P. Patel, K. Marsh, L. Carr, G. Nequist, Pharm. Res. 7 No. 9, S-165 (1990)
[428] H. Junginger, Pharm. Ind. 39, 498 (1977)
[429] N. Kaneniwa, A. Ikekawa, Chem. Pharm. Bull. 23, 2973–2986 (1975)
[430] N. Kaneniwa, A. Ikekawa, M. Sumi, a) Chem. Pharm. Bull. 26, 2734–2743 (1978); b) Chem. Pharm. Bull. 26, 2744–2758 (1978)
[431] I. Korner, R. Voigt, Pharmazie 33, 809 (1978)
[432] T. Sato, M. Ishiwata, S. Nemoto, H. Yamaguchi, T. Kobayasi, K. Sekiguchi, Y. Tsuda, Yakuzaigaku 49, 70–77 (1989)
[433] S. Leucuta, R. Pop, Clujul Med. 55, 60 (1982)
[434] Y. Nozawa, T. Mizumoto, F. Higashide, Yakuzaigaku 44, 134–140 (1984)
[435] Y. Nozawa, T. Mizumoto, F. Higashide, Pharm. Ind. 48, 967 (1986)
[436] Y. Nozawa, T. Taniyama, Yakuzaigaku 47, 197–203 (1987)
[437] R. Jachowicz, Int. J. Pharm. 35, 1 (1987)
[438] K. Kigasawa, K. Maruyama, M. Tanaka, O. Koyama, K. Watabe, Yakugaku Zasshi 101, 723–732 (1981)
[439] DOS 3503.682, Farmitalia-Carlo Erba (1984)
[440] Patents, Farmitalia-Carlo Erba (1985), a) DE 3503.679; b) DE 3503.681
[441] N. Visavarungroj, J. P. Remon, Int. J. Pharm. 62, 125–131 (1990)
[442] M. F. Saettone, B. Giannaccini, S. Ravecca, F. La Marca, Pharmakokin. Europ. Congr. 2, 620–626 (1984) + Int. J. Pharm. 20, Nos. 1–2, 187–202 (1984)
[443] C. Bantman, Immex 1, 133–136 (1972)
[444] H. Coulhon, P. Prevot, Ouest Médical 30 No. 1–2, 51–55 (1977)
[445] J. Hartman, Rev. Franc. Gastro-Entér. Oct., 77–78 (1971)
[446] M. Cachin, M. Neuman,a) Hopital/Info. Thérap. 3, 28–32 (1971); b) Hopital/Info. Thérap. 4, 37–38 (1971)
[447] R. E. Jeanpierre, R. Dornier, F. Vicari, J. X. Laurent, Méd. C. D. 6 No. 7, 499–503 (1977)
[448] P. E. Robert, C. Brechot, Anal. Gastroént. Hépato. (Paris) 8 No. 3, 299–304 (1972)
[449] J. M. Boboc, Méd. et Hygiène 36, 1330 (1978)
[450] C. Barthélemy, H. Fraisse, Lyon Médical 244 No. 19, 381–382 (1980)
[451] J. Guerre, M. Neuman, Méd. C. D. 8 No. 7, 679–682 (1979)
[452] Y. Barre, Gaz. Hopitaux 10 Nov., 869–870 (1971)
[453] P. Morère, J.-P. Stain, G. Nouvet, Presse Méd. 79 No. 41, 1812–1813 (1971)
[454] J. Taranger, C. Taranger, Semaine Hopitaux Thérap. Dec. (1971) + Thérapeutique 47 No. 10, 895–897 (1971)
[455] D. Thassu, S. P. Vyas, Drug Dev. Ind. Pharm. 17 No. 4, 561–576 (1991)

[456] G. P. Agrawal, D. C. Bhatt, Indian J. Pharm. Sci. Jan. – Feb., 54–55 (1990)
[457] M. Meshali, Y. El-Said, K. Gabr, Mans. J. Pharm. Sci. 6 No. 5, 126–145 (1990)
[458] B. Selmeczi, Arch. Pharm. 307, 755–759 (1974)
[459] A. Stamm, C. Mathis, J. Pharm. Belg. 29 No. 4, 375–389 (1974)
[460] Standardzulassungen für Fertigarzneimittel, Text und Kommentar, Deutscher Apothekerverlag (Dec. 1988)
[461] Eur. patent 063.266 (1982) BASF AG
[462] GB patent 1.594.001 (1977)
[463] US patent 3,851,032 (1974) + DE 2.338.234 (1973) + GB patent 1.410.909 (1971) Sterling Inc.
[464] Z. Vincze, A. Kubinyi, Gyógyszerészet 22, 377–379 (1978)
[465] Eur. patent 0.080.862 (1985) Beecham Group
[466] Eur. patent 0.063.014 (1985) Sankyo Ltd
[467] Eur. patent 0.055.397 (1981) Bayer AG
[468] Eur. patent 0.376.917 (1989) Burghart, Wien
[469] US patent 3,608,070 (1971) Nouvel, Paris
[470] A. A. Badwan, A. Abu-Malooh et al., Eur. J. Pharm. Biopharm. 37 No. 3, 166–170 (1991)
[471] Eur. patent 0.068.450 (1982) Rentschler
[472] Eur. patent 0.204.596 (1986) Rhone-Poulenc Santé
[473] DE 3441.308 (1985) Egyt Gyógyszervegyészeti Gyár, Budapest
[474] C. Brossard, D. Lefort, D. Duchène, F. Puisieux, J. T. Carstensen, J. Pharm. Sci. 72 No. 2, 162–169 (1983)
[475] Eur. patent 240.904 (1987) BASF AG
[476] Eur. patent 240.906 (1987) BASF AG
[477] DE 3810.343 (Offenlegungsschrift, 1988) BASF AG
[478] DOS 2849.029 (1980) Kali-Chemie
[479] Pharmeuropa 15 No. 2, April 2003, 352–353
[480] J. P. Patel, K. Marsh, L. Carr, G. Nequist, Int. J. Pharm. 65, 195–200 (1990)
[481] S. B. Jayaswal, A. Sharma, K. V. Chikhalidar, Indian J. Pharm. Sci. Jan. – Feb., 79 (1990)
[482] Eur. patent 089.245 (1983) Inter-Yeda, Israel
[483] H. G. Kirstensen, P. Holm, A. Jaegerskou, T. Schaefer, Pharm. Ind. 46 No. 7, 763–767 (1984)
[484] A. J. Romero, G. Lukas, C. T. Rhodes, Pharm. Acta Helv. 66 No. 2, 34–43 (1991)
[485] D. Giron, Acta Pharm. Jugosl. 40, 90–157 (1990)
[486] J. Akbuga, Pharm. Ind. 53 No. 9, 857–860 (1991)
[487] 21 Code of Federal Regulations (USA), § 173.55, (April 1991)
[488] 21 Code of Federal Regulations (USA), § 173.50, (April 1991)
[489] Eur. patent 428.486, Sandoz AG (1991)
[490] Japanese patent 3169814 (1991) Nippon Yakuhin Kogy
[491] S. P. Vyas, P. J. Gogoi, S. K. Jain, Drug Dev. Ind. Pharm. 17 No. 8, 1041–1058 (1991)
[492] T. V. Orlova, L. A. Ivanova, Farmatsiya 40 No. 4, 32–37 (1991)

[493] D. Faroongsarng, G. E. Peck, Drug Dev. Ind. Pharm. 17 No. 18, 2439–2455 (1991)
[494] S. Polito, D. W. Lee, W. A. McArthur, Pacemaker Leads 2, 401–404 (1985)
[495] N. Kohri, H. Yatabe, K. Iseki, K. Miyazaki, Int. J. Pharm. 68, 255–264 (1991)
[496] R. L. Gupta, R. Kumar, A. K. Singla, Drug. Dev. Ind. Pharm. 17 No. 3, 463–468 (1991)
[497] Eur. Patent 0.429.187 (1989) Elan Corp.
[498] J. Sawicka, Pharmazie 46 No. 4, 276–278 (1991)
[499] D. M. Wyatt, Manuf. Chem. 62 No. 12, 20–23 (1991)
[500] S. M. Safwat, S. S. Tous, M. M. Mohamed, Pharm. Ind. 53 No. 12, 1144–1150 (1991)
[501] M.-C. Etienne et al., J. Pharm. Sci. 80 No. 12, 1130–1132 (1991)
[502] G. Zoni, V. Lazzeretti, Boll. Chim. Farm. 106, 872–881 (1967)
[503] Z. T. Chowhan, A. A. Amaro, J. T. H. Ong, J. Pharm. Sci 81 No. 3, 290–294 (1992)
[504] A. Martini, C. Torricelli, R. De Ponti, Int. J. Pharm. 75, 141–146 (1991)
[505] DD 295 986 (1991) Bayer AG
[506] Eur. Patent 0.474.098 (1991) Senju
[507] US-Patent 4,874,690 (1989) Cryopharm
[508] F. Guillaume, A. M. Guyot-Hermann et al., Drug. Dev. Ind. Pharm. 18 No. 8, 811–827 (1992)
[509] Int. Patent WO 92/00730 (1990) Farcon
[510] C. Remuñán, M. J. Bretal, A. Nuñez, J. L. Vila Jato, Int. J. Pharm. 80, 151–159 (1992)
[511] R. Anders, H. P. Merckle, Int. J. Pharm. 49, 231–240 (1989)
[512] DE 4139.017 (1992) Egis
[513] F. A. Ismail, N. M. Khalafalla, S. A. Khalil, STP Pharm. Sci. 2 No. 4, 342–346 (1992)
[514] S. C. Mandal, S. C. Chattaraj, S. K. Goshal, Research + Ind. 37 No. 9, 168–170 (1992)
[515] L. Guomei, F. Rongyin, L. Xuewei, L. Muliang, Acta Sci. Nat. Univ. Sunyatseni 31 No. 1, 123–127 (1992)
[516] US-Patent 5,122,370 (1991) ISP
[517] US-Patent 5,084,276 (1990) Abbott
[518] Y. Nozaki, M. Kakumoto, M. Ohta, K. Yukimatsu, Drug Dev. Ind. Pharm. 19 No. 1+2, 221–275 (1993)
[519] P. K. Chakrabarti, D. J. Khodape, S. Bhattacharya, S. R. Naik, Ind. J. Pharm. Sci. 54 No. 3, 107–109 (1992)
[520] T. Nagai, K. Takayama, Proceedings 2nd Int. Symp. on Povidone, Lexington, 222–235 (1987)
[521] S. P. Vyas, S. Ramchandraiah, C. P. Jain, S. K. Jain, J. Microencaps. 9 No. 3, 347–355 (1992)
[522] G. Singh, S. N. Sharma, U. V Banakar, Acta Pharm. 42, 225–230 (1992)
[523] V. Vilivalam, Ch. M. Adeyeye, a. Pharm. Research 9/10, S-158 (1992); b. J. Microencaps. 11 No. 4, 455–470 (1994)

[524] M. del Pilar Buera, G. Levi, M. Karel, Biotech. Prog. 8, 144–148 (1992)
[525] J. Akbuga, K. Ermantas, Pharmazie 47 No. 8, 644–645 (1992)
[526] Eur. Patent 0.508.311 (1992) Mack
[527] C. W. Symecko, A. J. Romero, C. T. Rodes, Drug Dev. Ind. Pharm. 19 No. 10, 1131–1141 (1993)
[528] D. Vojnovic, F. Rubessa, N. Bogata, A. Mrhar, J. Microencaps. 10 No. 1, 89–99 (1993)
[529] DE 4211 883 (1992) Desitin
[530] K. Y. Paik, Dissertation Stevens Institute of Technologie, USA and Dissertation Abstracts Int. 52 No. 7 (1992)
[531] J. Kerc, N. Mohar, S. Srcic, B. Koflar, Acta Pharm. 43, 113–120 (1993)
[532] US-Patent 5,225,204 (1991)
[533] S. M. Safwat, S. T. P. Pharma Sci. 3 No. 4, 339–345 (1993)
[534] M. S. Gordon, Drug Dev. Ind. Pharm. 20 No. 1, 11–29 (1994)
[535] S. P. Vyas, C. P. Jain, S. Gupta, A. Uppadbayay, Drug Dev. Ind. Pharm. 20 No. 1, 101–110 (1994)
[536] S. G. Otabekova et al., Eksp. Klin. Farmakol. 56 No. 6, 50–52 (1993)
[537] S. Torrado et al., Proceed. Int. Symp. Contr. Release 20, 372–373 (1993)
[538] H. C. Meyer, J. B. Mielck, Eur. J. Pharm. Biopharm. 40, Suppl., 14 S (1994)
[539] S. C. Mandal, M. Bhattacharyya, S. K. Ghosal, Drug Dev. Ind. Pharm. 20 No. 11, 1933–1941 (1994)
[540] C-H. Liu et al., Drug Dev. Ind. Pharm. 20 No. 11, 1911–1922 (1994)
[541] N. Pourkavoos, G. E. Peck, Pharm. Res. 10 No. 8, 1212–1218 (1993)
[542] G. Bettinetti, P. Nura, Drug Dev. Ind. Pharm. 20 No. 8, 1353–1366 (1994)
[543] D. S. Desai, B. A. Rubitski, J. S. Bergum, S. A. Varia, Int. J. Pharm. 110 No. 3, 257–265 (1994) and Pharm. Res. 10 No. 10, S-142 (1993)
[544] N. Sinchalpanid, A. Nitrevej, J. Pharm. Sci. 20 No. 2, 33–39 (1993)
[545] C. F. Cartheuser, V. Acuna, L. Martínez, A. Sacristán, J. A. Ortiz, Methods Find. Exp. Clin. Pharm. 16 Suppl. 1, 85 (1994)
[546] A. Gupta, S. Garg, R. K. Khar, Drug Dev. Ind. Pharm. 20 No. 3, 315–325 (1994)
[547] T. Sate, P. Venkitachalam, Drug Dev. Ind. Pharm. 20 No. 19, 3005–30014 (1994)
[548] M. Moneghini, D. Vojnovic, F. Rubessa, G. Zingone, Acta Tech. Legis Med. Vol. III, No. 3, 149–161 (1992)
[549] C.-H. Liu, S.-C. Chen, Y.-C. Lee, T. D. Sokoloski, M.-T. Sheu, Drug Dev. Ind. Pharm. 20 No. 11, 1911–1922 (1994)
[550] A. P. Simonelli, M. M. Meshali, H. Abd El-Gawad, H. M. Abdel-Aleem, K. E. Gabr, Pharm. Ind. 57 No. 1, 72–76 (1995)
[551] V. V. Boldyrev, T. P. Shakhtshneider, L. P. Burleva, V. A. Severtsev, Drug Dev. Ind. Pharm. 20 No. 6, 1103–1114 (1994)
[552] J. R. Pettis, B. A. Middleton, J. M. Cho, Pharm. Res. 11 No. 10, Suppl. S231 (1994)
[553] H. Ibrahim, E. Sallam, R. AbuDahab, M. Shubair, Pharm. Res. 11 No. 10, Suppl., S165 (1994)

[554] G. Zingone, F. Rubessa, S. T. P. Pharma Sci. 4 (2) 122–127 (1994)
[555] S.-J. Hwang et al., Int. J. Pharm. 116, 125–128 (1995)
[556] T. Loftsson, A. M. Siguroardottir, Eur. J. Pharm. Sci. No. 4, 297–301 (1994) + Int. J. Phar. 126, 73–78 (1995)
[557] K. Sekizaki, K. Danjo, H. Eguchi, Y. Yonezawa, H. Sunada, A. Otzuka, Chem. Pharm. Bull. 43 No. 6, 988–993 (1995)
[558] Canadian Patent 2,125,060 (Bausch & Lomb, 1994)
[559] Y. Lee, Y. W. Chien, Pharm. Res. 11 No. 10, Suppl., S300 (1994) + J. Contr. Release 37, 251–261 (1995)
[560] Internat. Patent WO 94/25008 (Procter & Gamble, 1994)
[561] T. K. Mandal, Drug Dev. Ind. Pharm. 21 No. 14,1683–1688 (1995)
[562] Eur. Patent 0 621 033 A1 (Greenfeed)
[563] W. Sawicki, S. Janicki, Farm. Pol. 51 No. 14, 599–603 (1995)
[564] N. Follonier, E. Doelker, E. T. Cole, J. Contr. Release 36, 243–250 (1995)
[565] E. Ochoa Machiste, P. Giunchedi, M. Setti, U. Conte, Int. J. Pharm. 126, 65–72 (1995)
[566] A. P. Simonelli, M. M Meshali et al., Mans. J. Pharm. Sci. 11 No.1, 16–34 (1995)
[567] N. A. Megrab, A. C. Williams, B. W. Barry, J. Contr. Release 36, 277–294 (1995)
[568] Y.-S. Sihn, L. Kirsch, Pharm. Res.12/9, S-145 (1995)
[569] J. G. Kesavan, G. E. Peck, Drug Dev. Ind. Pharm. 22 No. 3, 189–199 (1996)
[570] Y. Nozaki, K. Yukimatsu, T. Mayumi, STP Pharm. Sci. 6 No. 2, 134–141 (1996)
[571] W. Sawicki, K. Cal, S. Janicki, Farm. Pol. 52 No.10, 440–444 (1996)
[572] M. Iwata, H. Ueda, Drug Dev. Ind. Pharm. 22 No.11, 1161–1165 (1996)
[573] A. F. Brown, D. S. Jones, A. D. Woolfson, Eur. J. Pharm. Sci. 4 Suppl. S 176 (1996)
[574] D. S. Jones, A. D. Woolfson, J. Djokic, C. R. Erwin, Eur. J. Pharm. Sci. 4 Suppl. S 145 (1996)
[575] Int. Patent WO 96/22103 (Cheil Foods + Chem.1996)
[576] J. Kerc, S. Srcic, B. Kofler, Proceed. lnt. Symp. Contr. Rel. Bio. Mater., 24, 381–382 (1997)
[577] K. P. R. Chowdary, K. V. R. Murthy, Ch. D .S. Prasod, Indian Drugs 32 No.11, 537–541 (1995)
[578] M. M. Feldstein et al., Int. J. Pharm. 131, 229–242 (1996)
[579] South Africa Patent 43 7114 (1978)
[580] P. W. S. Heng, L. S. C. Wan, Y. T. F. Tan, Int. J. Pharm. 138, 57–66 (1996)
[581] N. K. Ebube et al., Drug Dev. Ind. Pharm. 22 No. 7, 561–567 (1996)
[582] B. K. Dubey, O. P. Katare, R. Sing, S. K. Jain, J. Derm. Sci. 10, 191–195 (1995)
[583] A. Ahuja, M. Dogra, S. P. Agarwal, Indian J. Pharm. Sci. 57 No.1, 26–30 (1995)
[584] P. J. Antony, N. M. Sanghavi, Drug Dev. Ind. Pharm. 23 No. 4, 413–415 (1997)
[585] V. Tantishaiyakul et al., Int. J. Pharm. 143, 59–66 (1996) + 181, 143-151 (1999)
[586] S. Torrado, S. Torrado, J. J. Torrado, R. Cadórniga, Int. J. Pharm. 140, 247–250 (1996)

[587] G. K. Jain, A. K. Sharma, S. S. Agrawal, Int. J. Pharm. 130, No. 2, 169–177 (1996)
[588] H. Akin, J. Heller, F. W. Harris, Polymer Reprint 38 No.1, 241–242 (1997)
[589] European Patent EP 0 626 843 B1 (SB, 1993)
[590] European Patent EP 0 781 550 A1 (Servier)
[591] M. F. L. Law, P. B. Deasy, Eur. J. Pharm. + Biopharm. 45, 57–65 (1998)
[592] E. J. Vining, A. C. Williams, B. W. Barry, J. Pharm. Pharmacol. 49/1, 81 (1997)
[593] Internat. Patent WO 97/23206 (3M, 1995)
[594] D. S. Jones, A. D. Woolfson, A. F. Brown, Pharm. Res.14 No. 4, 450–457 (1997)
[595] E. Sallam, H. Ibrahim, R. Abu Dahab, M. Shubair, E. Khalil, Drug. Dev. Ind. Pharm. 24 (6), 501–507 (1998)
[596] T. Murakami, M. Yoshioka et al., J. Pharm. Pharmacol. 50, 49–54 (1998)
[597] G.van den Mooter, P. Augustijns, N. Blaton, R. Kinget, Int. J. Pharm. 164 No. 1–2, 567–580 (1998)
[598] Y. Morita, H. Saino, K. Tojo, Biol. Pharm. Bul. 21 No. 1, 72–75 (1998)
[599] P. Rama Rao, P. V. Diwan, Drug Dev. Ind. Pharm. 24 (4), 327–336 (1998)
[600] C. D. Zanetti, O. Quattrocci, R. Costanzo, SAFYBI (Argentine) 32 (87) 52–60 (1992)
[601] D.Zupancic Bozic, F. Vrecer, K. Kozjek, Eur. J. Pharm. Sci. 5, 163–169 (1997)
[602] R. Shettigar, A. V. Damle, Indian J. Pharm. Sci. 58 No. 5, 179–183 (1996)
[603] P. B. Deasy, M. F. L. Law, Int. J. Pharm. 148, 201–209 (1997)
[604] M. C. Tros de llarduya, C. Martin, M. M. Goñi, M. C.Martínez-Ohárriz, Drug Dev. Ind. Pharm. 24 (3), 295–300 (1998)
[605] E. A. Pariente, G. de la Garoullaye, Méd. C. D. 23 No.3, 193–199 (1994)
[606] H. Y. Karasulu, G. Ertan, T. Güneri, Eur. J. Drug Metab. Pharmacokinet. 18, 108–114 (1993) + 21 No.1, 27–31 (1996)
[607] P. Sancin, L.Rodríguez, C. Cavallari et al., Farm. Vestn. 48, Spec. Issue, 256–257 (1997)
[608] Russ. Patent 2060031 (Onkologitcheskii Nautchnyi Tsentr, 1996)
[609] L + S AG, Endotoxin Validation Report, 10. August 1998
[610] S. K. El-Arini, H. Leuenberger, Pharm. Acta Helv. 73, 89–94 (1998)
[611] Europa Patent 0 317 281 B1 (1992, Wellcome)
[612] W. Sawicki, S. Janicki, S.T.P. Pharma Sci. 8(2), 107–111 (1998)
[613] M. Moneghini, A. Carcano, G. Zingone, B. Perissutti, Int. J. Pharm. 175, 177–183 (1998)
[614] P. Martínez, M.M. Goñi et al., Eur. J. Drug Metab. Pharmacokinet. 23 No. 2, 113–117 (1998)
[615] V. Bühler, "Generic Drug Formulations", BASF Fine Chemicals, Ludwigshafen, Germany, 4th edition 2001
[616] R. Thilbert, C.R. Dalton, A.-R. Moallemi, D. Projean, B.C. Hancock, Pharm. Res. Suppl. 14, 11, S-482 (1997)
[617] S.-C. Shin, I.-J. Oh, Y.-B. Lee, H.-K. Choi, J.-S. Choi, Int. J. Pharm. 175, 17–24 (1998)
[618] G. Petersen, H. G. Kristensen, Drug Dev. Ind. Pharm. 25(1), 69–74 (1999)
[619] K. Kreft, B. Kozamernik, U. Urleb, Int. J. Pharm. 177, 1–6 (1999)

[620] Y.T.F. Tan, L.S.C. Wan, P.W.S. Heng, S.T.P. Pharma Sciences 8(3) 149–153 (1998)
[621] Int. Patent WO 97/49437 (Astra) 1997
[622] US Patent 5,703, 111 (Bristol-Myers Squibb) 1997
[623] M. Oechsner, S. Keipert, Eur. J. Pharm. Biopharm. 47, 113–118 (1999)
[624] Eur. Patent EP 0 780 121 A1 (Chauvin) 1996
[625] Int. Patent WO 98/05312 (Ascent Pediadrics) 1996
[626] US Patent 5,811,130 (Pfizer) 1998
[627] D.S. Jones, C.R. Irwin, A.D. Woolfson, J. Diokic, V. Adams, J. Pharm. Sci. 88(6) 592–598 (1999)
[628] Int. Patent WO 97/26895 (Komer) 1997
[629] S. Hülsmann, T. Backensfeld, S. Keitel, R. Bodmeier, Eur. J. Pharm. Biopharm. 49, 237–242 (2000)
[630] E. Khalil, S. Najjar, A. Sallam, Drug Dev. Ind. Pharm. 26(4) 375–381 (2000)
[631] Pharmeuropa 10(3) Sept. 1998, 413–415
[632] D.S. Jones et al., J. Contr. Release 67, 357–368 (2000)
[633] Int. Patent WO 00/09096 (Nanosystems, USA) 1999
[634] T. Nabekura, Y. Ito, H. Cai, M. Terao, R. Hori, Biol. Pharm. Bull. 23 (5), 616–620 (2000)
[635] M. Moneghini, A. Carcano, B. Perissutti, F. Rubessa, Pharm. Dev. Tech. 5 (2), 297–301 (2000)
[636] V. lannucelli, G. Coppi, E. Leo, F. Fontana, M. T. Bernabei, Drug Dev. lnd. Pharm. 26 (6) 595–603 (2000)
[637] G. Shlieout, Proc. 3rd World Meeting APV/APGI, Berlin, 3/6 April 2000
[638] P. de la Torre, Su. Torrado, Sa. Torrado, Chem. Pharm. Bull. 47 (11) 1629–1633 (1999)
[639] O. Shakoor, D.F. Bain, N.C. Duguid, C. R. Park, J. Pharm. Pharmacol. 51 (Supplement), 286 (1999)
[640] R. Eyjolfsson, Pharmazie 54 (12) 945 (1999)
[641] C.R. Park, D.F. Bain, D.L. Munday, P. Ramluggun, O. Shakoor, J. Pharm. Pharmacol. 52 (Supplement), 303 (2000)
[642] K.P.R. Chowdary, S. Srinivasa Rao, Drug Dev. Ind. Pharm. 26 (11), 1207–1211 (2000)
[643] G. van den Mooter, M. Wuyts et al., Eur. J. Pharm. Sci. 12, 261–269 (2001)
[644] Z. Musko, K. Pintye Hodi et al., Eur. J. Pharm. Biopharm. 51 No. 2, 143–146 (2001)
[645] C. Valenta, T. Dabic, Drug Dev. lnd. Pharm. 27 No. 1, 57–62 (2001)
[646] F. Zhang, J.W. MacGinity, Drug Dev. Ind. Pharm. 26 No. 9, 931–942 (2000)
[647] E.Draganoiu, M.Andheria, A.Sakr, Pharm.Ind. 63, No. 6, 624–629 (2001)
[648] E.Draganoiu, A.Sakr, Brit.Pharm.Conference 2001 Abstracts, 136 (2001)
[649] Z.J.Shao, M.I.Farooqi, S.Diaz, A.K.Krisna, N.A.Muhamed, Pharm.Dev.Tech. 6(2), 247–254 (2001)
[650] J.M.Bultmann, Proceedings 4th World Meeting APGI/APV, Florence, April 2002, 175–176

[651] F.Wöll, P.Kleinebudde, Proceedings 4th World Meeting APGI/APV, Florence, April 2002, 159–160
[652] US Pharmacopeial Forum Vol. 28 No. 3, 948–951 (May–June 2002)
[653] A.Moroni, Pharm.Technol. 25, Suppl., 8–24 (2001)
[654] S.Schiermeier, P.C.Schmidt, Eur. J. Pharm. Sci. 15, 295–305 (2002)
[655] US Patent 5 464 632 (Prographarm, F) 1995
[656] M.A.Elliott, S.J.Ford, A.A.Walker, R.H.J.Hargreaves, G.W.Halbert, J. Pharm. Pharmacol.54, 487–492 (2002)
[657] P.Sharma, V.Hamsa, S.T.P.Pharma Sci. 11 (4) 275–281 (2001)
[658] J.-Y.Fang, K.-C.Sung, O.Y.-P.Hu, H.-Y.Chen, Drug Research 51 (I), 408–413 (2001)
[659] H.Afrasiabi Garekani, A.Ghazi, K.Pharm.Pharmacol. 54, Suppl., S92 (2002)
[660] A.Roda, L.Sabatini, M.Mirasoli, M.Baraldini, E.Roda, Int.J.Pharm. 241, 165–172 (2002)
[661] Z.Muskó, J.Bajdik, K.Pintye-Hódi et al., Pharm.Ind. 64, No. 11, 1194–1198 (2002)
[662] U. Shah, L. Augsburger, Pharm. Dev. Tech. 6 (1) 39–51 (2001)

7 Alphabetical index